Dear future physician,

You are about to embar[k on a journey that is both rewarding] and challenging. Since you are in your first year of medical school, we wanted to introduce you to the Medical Association of Georgia (MAG) – which has been the leading voice for physicians in the state since 1849.

MAG's mission is to, "Enhance patient care and the health of the public by advancing the art and science of medicine and by representing physicians and patients in the policy making process."

With more than 7,800 members, MAG is an advocate for physicians in every specialty and practice setting in the state. MAG also represents medical students in Georgia.

We believe that we can protect and preserve one of the best health care systems in the world if we stand united as a profession. That is why we encourage you to take an active role in the policy-making process in the state early in your career. Doing so means that you will be taking an active role in determining your fate as a physician in Georgia.

Sir William Osler, M.D., who was one of the founders of Johns Hopkins School of Medicine, said that, "You cannot afford to stand aloof from your professional colleagues in any place. Join their associations, mingle in their meetings, giving of the best of your talents."

With this in mind, we encourage you to go to www.mag.org or call 678.303.9261 to join MAG. The cost is just $5 for all four years.

We also encourage you to become active in MAG's Medical Student Section, which will give you the opportunity to exchange information and ideas with your peers across the state – as well as have a unified voice in organized medicine in Georgia.

We applaud long-time MAG member Barry Silverman, M.D. — who has been caring for his patients in Atlanta for nearly 50 years — for taking the initiative to write this important book. We would also like to thank Dr. Silverman for making this book available to every first-year medical student in the state for free. It's a great resource – one that offers some great wisdom and advice as you prepare for your career as a physician.

Finally, we should never forget that the foundation for the American health care system is the physician-patient relationship. The clinical side of the equation is obviously important. But we must also remember that we are often interacting with people when they are at their most vulnerable – so it is equally important to tend to their emotional needs and calm their fears while we heal their bodies. We believe that the best doctors are those whose bedside manner is humane, compassionate, empathetic, and supportive.

There isn't a more important, rewarding profession than medicine – so congratulations and best wishes as you embark on your journey to become a physician.

John S. Harvey, M.D.
President, Medical Association of Georgia

Jack M. Chapman Jr., M.D.
President, MAG Foundation

Praises for:
Your Doctors' Manners Matter

Good manners are important in every area of our lives, but as the authors argue, no more so than in our relations with doctors and medical staff. The authors note a deterioration of manners in society in general—especially in the medical field—and insist that good manners also make good medicine. Illustrated with moving vignettes of patients and their doctors, *Your Doctors' Manners Matter* advises patients on what to expect from doctors in office and hospital settings and how to effectively communicate with them. The book makes for insightful reading for patients and doctors alike.

– Anthony Grooms, author of *Bombingham*

It is very important and timely and of value to patients and I think health professionals and their staff.

– Thomas J. Murray, OC, MD, FRCP © MACP, LLD(HON), DSc(HON), FRCP(LON)

Saul Adler adds his name to the list of good doctors who have become good writers. His vision of courteous service in health care is just what the doctor ordered.

– Roy Peter Clark, author of *Writing Tools* and *How to Write Short*

YOUR DOCTORS' MANNERS MATTER

YOUR DOCTORS' MANNERS MATTER:
Better Health through Civility in the Doctor's Office and in the Hospital

Barry Silverman, MD and Saul Adler, MD

BOOKLOGIX®

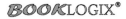

Alpharetta, GA

All rights reserved. No part of this book may be reproduced or transmitted in any form or by any means, electronic or mechanical, including photocopying, recording, or any information storage and retrieval system, without permission in writing from the publisher. For more information address Permissions Department, 1264 Old Alpharetta Rd., Alpharetta, GA 30005 or permissions@booklogix.com.

Use of *The New Consultation: Developing Doctor-Patient Communication* is with permission of Oxford University Press.

Copyright © 2014 by Barry Silverman and Saul Adler

Paperback Edition January 2014

ISBN: 978-1-61005-447-8

Library of Congress Control Number: 2013921354

(For information about bulk purchases, please contact the publisher.)

10 9 8 7 6 5 4 3 2   0 1 2 0 1 4

Printed in the United States of America

∞This paper meets the requirements of ANSI/NISO Z39.48-1992 (Permanence of Paper)

To Martha and Rosalyn

"I observe the physician with the same diligence as he the disease."

– John Donne, 1573–1631

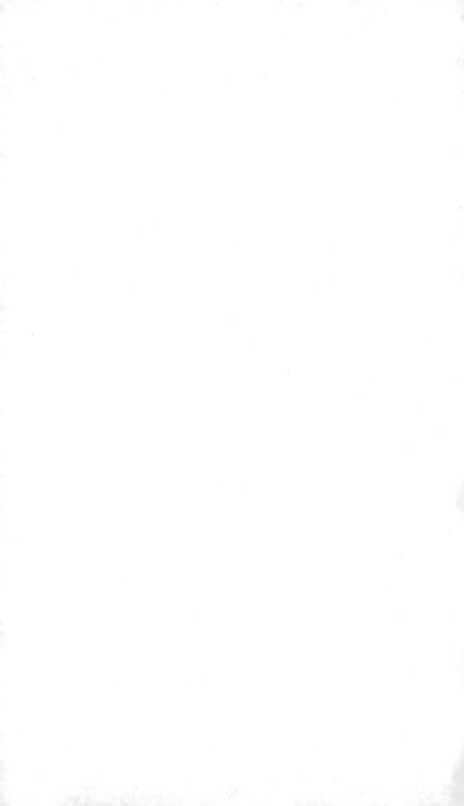

Contents

Acknowledgments	xiii
Introduction	xv

Section One Why It's Nice to Be Nice

Chapter One Manners, Medicine, and Morals	3
Chapter Two Compassion and Communication	27
Chapter Three Behavior of the Effective Physician	41

Section Two Finding the Right Doctor

Chapter Four The Office Consultation	71
Chapter Five The Hospital Experience	103
Chapter Six At the Pediatrician: A Teachable Moment	157
Conclusion Some Parting Advice	173
References	179
About the Authors	185

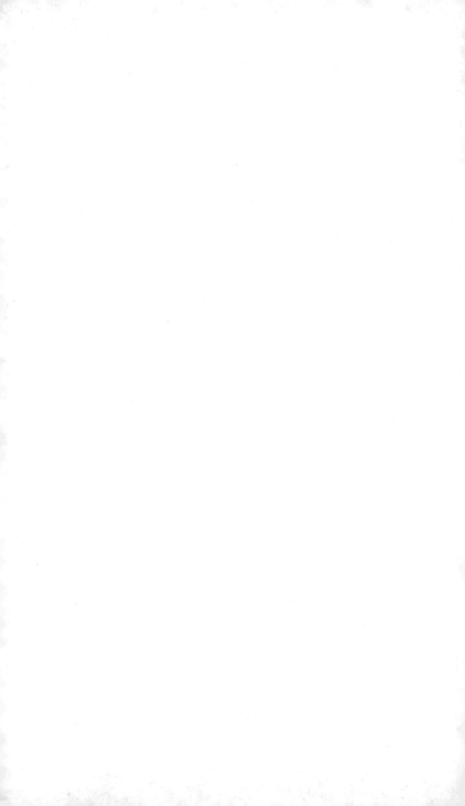

Acknowledgments

We thank the many physicians, nurses, and patients who have contributed to the contents of this book by their critique of our behavior, both positively and otherwise. We also thank those physicians and patients who show grace under pressure. They stand as beacons in the dark of despair and disarray.

We thank the early readers of our book, the members of the Sunday Writers Group, Brenda Ledford, Sussan Sutphen, MD, and Professor Todd Campbell. Their critiques were models of mannerliness. Thank you to Judi Kanne, RN, BSN, BA for her extensive review of several chapters, and to Felice Adler, MD for her review of the chapter on pediatrics. They both offered many good suggestions. Any omission is of our doing.

We would like to offer a special appreciation to the late Mark Silverman, MD whose advice and counsel was critical to the creation of this book.

Barry Silverman, MD
Saul Adler, MD

Introduction

The life of a sick person can be shortened not only by the acts, but by the words and manner of the physician. It is therefore, a sacred duty to guard himself carefully in this respect, and to avoid all things which have a tendency to discourage the patient and to depress his spirits...It must be admitted that these rules are not infrequently violated. Does it follow that these rules are useless? Certainly not. The fact only proves that knowledge of rules does not always secure their observance... Prescribed rules of conduct are of use by giving distinctness and force to popular sentiment. Moreover, the knowledge of rules affects the conduct of those who, not devoid of rectitude, pursue the wrong because they do not know the right. Rules thus tend to nullify the temptations and specious pleadings of apparent self-interest.[1]

– Austin Flint, Sr., MD, 1883
Professor of Medicine and Founder of the Medical
School at Bellevue Hospital in New York City

Have you ever visited a physician who is uncommunicative, arrogant, or sarcastic? Or perhaps the doctor is respectful, but the office staff is unfriendly or uncooperative and the nurses are rude or abrupt. When you do finally get to see the doctor, your time together is all too short, and yet your consultation is interrupted by a beeper, cell phone, or the nurse. Maybe your doctor is habitually late for appointments and overbooked, or you have to sit forever before you are ushered into the exam room, only to wait half-naked or in a flimsy paper gown.

These are just a few of the problems patients face in a doctor's office. It gets worse in the hospital where you might experience unfriendly admitting clerks, long waits, insolent or sharp-tongued nurses, unkempt and abrasive staff, cold tables, hard uncomfortable chairs, and long periods where you are left alone, wondering if you have been forgotten. And yet, all this is nothing compared to the treatment you get at the hands of the third-party insurers who seem to reject any semblance of customer service.

The healthcare industry is moving against the tide in our consumer-oriented economy. Hotels, restaurants, sports arenas, and department stores recognize that courteous, friendly service and good manners make for a successful business, while medical establishments seem to cling to behavior that lies somewhere between uncivil and downright rude. While indifferent or rude behavior in healthcare may seem a trivial issue, a great deal of evidence, both anecdotally and in the research literature, indicates that good manners and professional behavior at every level of healthcare results in better outcomes.

During my forty years of practice, most spent as the director of cardiology at a large community hospital, I have witnessed a gradual change in the professional

Your Doctors' Manners Matter

behavior of doctors, nurses, and allied health personnel. Before his untimely death in 2008, I frequently discussed this issue with my older brother, Mark Silverman, a Professor of Medicine at Emory University School of Medicine and director of the Fuqua Heart Institute at Piedmont Hospital in Atlanta, Georgia. We identified rude professional behavior as one of the problems we encounter in caring for our patients. We came to appreciate that poor medical outcomes are rarely based on a lack of knowledge and most certainly not a lack of caring, but often are a result of bad manners and occasionally outright boorish behavior. Such conduct in a social setting is annoying and leads to social avoidance of the offender. In a medical setting, it leads to mistakes, causes anxiety, prolongs patient recovery, and influences patient dissatisfaction with the medical care received and caregiver dissatisfaction with the work they are doing. While true malpractice is rare, we identified behavior problems on an almost daily basis that had the potential of causing a poor but preventable medical outcome, a tragedy for the patient and a potential lawsuit for the caregivers.

When I was invited to lecture on the subject, the feedback and questions that followed indicated that poor manners and rude behavior are all too common in medicine. In 2005, I wrote a pamphlet to use as a handout at the lectures. It included lists of suggestions for doctors to improve communication with the patient at the bedside, with nurses on the wards, and with consulting physicians. The pamphlet was not unlike the checklists recommended by Atul Gawande in his book *The Checklist Manifesto: How to Get Things Right*.[2] This book, *Your Doctors' Manners Matter*, was written in collaboration with Dr. Saul Adler and arose out of the conversations with my late brother and my lectures.

Patients who are confronted with bad manners will recognize a need for an instruction manual in professional behavior, manners, and decorum. Why direct the book to you, the patient, and not to physicians? There are physicians who are unaware of either the effect of their behavior on their patients, or even that they are acting in an inappropriate way. We can imagine their responses. Possibly something like "Who are these guys anyway?" Then in quick succession and as the age gap increases, "Elitist. Outdated. Archaic." Or perhaps we will hear the remark our teenage children frequently threw at us: "It's different now," implying that the rules have changed. Therefore, an instruction manual in manners for the profession might be received in a less than enthusiastic manner.

To our knowledge, not a single medical school offers a formal course in professional and social behavior. Apparently it's a given that twenty-five-year-old women and men acquire these social graces well before they become medical students, and any instruction in the specifics of proper professional behavior at the bedside is learned by example from the senior physician and professor.[3] That is the tradition. The tradition is not working.

Although more and more of our medical school professors are first-rate scientists, many do not have extensive hands-on patient care experience. In the book *Learning to Heal: The Development of American Medical Education,* Kenneth Ludmerer describes how our medical schools have changed in the past 100 years.[4] Where previously students received instruction from clinicians in private practice, now senior professors and other faculty have little direct patient care experience. Medical students learn their bedside manners from other students, young residents, and junior faculty. Their exposure to a senior, experienced clinician is brief and increasingly rare. Methods of interacting with the patient and family that served well in the past—before the huge technological innovations of the past thirty years—are ignored, considered irrelevant, out of date, or just not possible in our present healthcare system.

The Patient as Master

Of course, the authors welcome the physician and medical student as readers, but our hope is you, the patient, armed with reasonable expectations of behavior and with the authority of an educated consumer, can act as an instructor of sorts for the profession. You can reinforce excellent behavior and voice polite requests for a fair accommodation of your needs when appropriate. This will create a two-way street. As the doctor teaches you ways to better care for yourself, you can, through implication and innuendo, impart to the doctor and the medical staff your expectations of their behavior.

You have certain expectations concerning your physician's behavior. You expect the physician to listen. If in the hospital, you should be told when rounds are planned. The physician should be open to schedule conferences with your family. You expect to learn the results of laboratory studies in a timely fashion. These are good manners, yes, but are also indicative of a doctor who has accepted a commitment concerning your welfare.

Diane Payne's experience offers a real-life example of the effects of doctors acting poorly on a patient's family. Her story is described in an article "Crisis in Medicine" appearing in a 2005 issue of *Newsweek* magazine. Diane's husband developed a sudden illness and died after thirty-eight days in the intensive care unit of one of Atlanta's largest and most respected suburban hospitals. In the story, she describes the behavior of the doctors who cared for her husband:

> If you miss the doctor, don't expect him to call you later with a report on how your loved one is doing. And forget about calling him at his office. Some receptionists won't even pretend to deliver

a request to the doctor for a phone call from anyone other than a patient's ICU nurse. To make matters worse there isn't just one doctor, my husband had eight, not uncommon with critically ill patients.[5]

Polite behavior in the medical office and the hospital not only improves the care patients receive, the behavior of the doctor and staff is a reflection of the moral underpinnings of their commitment to their patients and their profession. Judith Martin, the syndicated columnist who writes as Miss Manners—an authority on the rules of etiquette—authored an article for the Proceedings of the American Philosophical Society making just that point. She wrote: "Morality and etiquette form a single, albeit highly complex—and by no means conflict-free—system of rules for the governance of social conduct."[6]

Manners-Based Medicine

The term "evidence-based medicine" refers to the use of information obtained by the scientific method to determine the best medical treatment for a particular patient. When we use the term manners-based medicine, we mean interpersonal behavior that expresses the moral principles underlying medicine. They are respect for human dignity, courtesy, acting to benefit the patient, causing no intentional harm, treating the patient with justice, and dedication to medical service. However, manners-based medicine goes beyond doctor and patient interaction. Manners-based medicine can be applied to interactions between doctors and nurses, technicians, assistants, and administrators, each individual involved in healthcare acting in a polite and well-mannered fashion that signals he or she recognizes the dignity of the other person.

In what follows, we will not present a code of etiquette meant to distinguish the boorish from the elite, the newcomer from the established, and the favored from the invisible. Rather, we will demonstrate from our observations, experience, and interviews how healthcare workers who conduct themselves in the office, hospital, and clinic in a manner that communicates to patients and each other an understanding of the other person's humanity will get better health results. We will show you how to identify by their manners those doctors and nurses who have superior patient compliance and outcomes and greater patient satisfaction. Not coincidentally, these are the doctors and nurses most satisfied with their chosen profession.

In this book, you will read stories of patient care, some funny, others sad, and still others frustrating, that demonstrate how polite behavior can improve medical care and how rude behavior or indifferent attitudes can be harmful, even life-threatening. You will learn steps you as a patient can take to improve manners and communication as well as advice on how, when confronted by hurtful and harmful behavior, you can respond. As we explain to you, the patient, how to identify the best doctors and nurses by their behavior, the careful reader will note the implications for physicians and nurses on office and bedside behavior designed to improve patient outcomes.

Each chapter contains at least one patient narrative that illustrates the points we are trying to make. Names of patients and institutions are fictitious, although the stories are real. At the end of each chapter are a series of bullet points summarizing the main issues discussed in the chapter.

Those who know us might be tempted to point fingers, claiming that neither of us has always been perfectly behaved. We admit it. There are times when, without offering excuses, we have been guilty of transgressing the boundaries of good manners. We have learned from experience. Looking back, we can see where we and others went astray. (We admonish the finger-pointers; it is bad manners to do so.)

We are very sympathetic to reactive misbehavior, the response to passive-aggressive behavior and deliberate misbehavior calculated to incite negative reactions. Any of our colleagues who read this book will be alerted to potential pitfalls and we hope avoid reactive misbehavior.

We hope to show how the practice of good manners demonstrates concern for each other and marks the compassionate caregiver. Adopting the practice of everyday good manners in the medical office, clinic, and hospital can decrease costs by improving diagnostic accuracy with good listening techniques, foster trust by focusing attention on the patient, and improve patient follow-through by exhibiting compassion and empathy. Further, appropriate behavior among colleagues and toward patients will go a long way toward reducing the dissatisfaction many healthcare providers and patients struggle with on a daily basis.

In our experience, medical errors frequently result from physicians and healthcare personnel who are inconsiderate and communicate poorly. The Institute of Medicine estimates 100,000 deaths occur a year in hospitals because of medical errors; some a result of careless, rude, or inconsiderate behavior. We believe such errors can be reduced or eliminated with little cost to patient or doctor by practicing medicine in a polite and agreeable manner.

Even the most educated patient is unable to personally evaluate medical skills. But certain behavior characteristics indicate a healthcare worker who is capable of empathy and caring, and one who takes pride in his or her profession. The patient who is knowledgeable about the behavior of the respectful physician will be able to identify the most effective

Your Doctors' Manners Matter

doctors and may be able to improve the behavior of those medical professionals who do not yet understand how a conscientious display of civility, respect, and empathy are indispensable tools of their profession.

How to Use this Book

This book is divided into two sections. In Section One we explain in general terms why we believe, through our observations and experience, your doctors' good manners will go far to improve your health. In this section, we also draw on popular culture, philosophy, and a short history of the loss of medical manners to help justify our argument that good manners on the part of healthcare workers are not only worth the time and effort in terms of your health, but are a matter of morality.

In Section Two, we are very specific about what you will observe in those doctors' offices and hospitals that will deliver superior care to you. If you are concerned about your doctor, or if you are in the process of deciding where to get your medical care, you might go to Section Two first.

Barry Silverman, MD, FACC
Saul Adler, MD, FAAP
Atlanta, Georgia
July 18, 2013

SECTION ONE
Why It's Nice to Be Nice

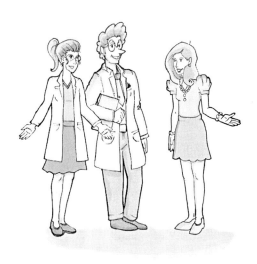

Chapter One

Manners, Medicine, and Morals

Manners are of more importance than laws. Upon them, in a great measure, the laws depend. The law touches us but here and there and now and then. Manners are what vex or soothe, corrupt or purify, exalt or debase, barbarize or refine us, by a constant, steady, uniform, insensible operation, like that of the air we breathe in. They give their whole form and colour to our lives. According to their quality, they aid morals, they supply them, or they totally destroy them.

– Edmund Burke, 1729–1797

Manners versus Etiquette

You bare your body voluntarily, prepared to suffer poking and prodding into crevices and crannies where few others have likely ventured, or bravely suffer the insertion of sharp and painful instruments where none belong—and you pay for the experience. This is not a bizarre initiation rite, and you have not stumbled into a sadistic terrorist den. You're in your doctor's office, and you might suppose the medical staff, with whom you have entrusted the integrity of still-attached body parts, to exhibit sympathy and just a little deference for your bravery. Furthermore, it is not unreasonable to expect courtesy at least comparable to your bank teller, responsible only for your money, or the barista at your coffee house, accountable for the foam on your latte. But often the medical staff in the office or in the hospital exhibits rude, churlish behavior, justifying their bad attitude with excuses: they are rushed, overbooked, dealing with emergencies, or underpaid by third parties. They are not responsible for their attitude—it's all a result of circumstances beyond control. Besides, the office manager might say—if you have the temerity to complain—the doctor is the best in town and it doesn't really matter if he is rushed, or if she is frequently interrupted by phone calls, or if the computer screen gets more face time than you. What really matters is that you will get well.

Not so. Brusque and often rude behavior is not merely a question of incivility—good manners can make a difference in the quality of care a patient receives.

Your Doctors' Manners Matter

We are all supposed to act in a civil and courteous manner, having been taught lessons in manners and proper behavior since early childhood. However, if the number of books and articles complaining about and offering advice on interpersonal behavior is any indication, additional instruction is needed. The problem is modern society looks on lists of complex rules—etiquette—as a gate designed and erected by the privileged to exclude the unwanted and unschooled.

The terms manners and etiquette are often used interchangeably, but they are different. Manners are a description of social behavior. We learn our manners from our parents and teachers by example, instruction, and training, or we mimic the behavior of our friends and role models. Bad manners might reflect on childhood training, deliberate contrariness, or social mimicking.

Every society has rules defining the norms of social behavior. These are the rules of etiquette dealing with table manners, dress codes for work and social events, and behavior in school, on the athletic fields, in the office, and for every social situation.

Rules of etiquette seem always to be under attack. Each new generation views the behavior of their elders as archaic and stuffy, and rules of behavior and those who advance them as unnecessary tools. In the Victorian era, complex rules of etiquette were used to separate social groups, advance snobbery, describe the way the best people were to behave, and distinguish the so-called well-bred from the common man. In a society where new wealth made possible by commerce and industrialization caused ancestral barriers to crumble, social rules of etiquette limited the elite class to the well-bred. If you didn't know the rules you weren't admitted into the game, but if you followed the rules you could hide your background.

Up until the 1950s, rules of etiquette were often complex, restrictive, and unreasonable lists for everything from how to enter and leave an elevator, when a man should lift his hat and who should be first through a doorway. The rules were designed to preserve the social stature of those born to wealth and position, protect the power of a male-dominated authority, and exclude those without the time, training, or desire to master their complexities. For many, the rules of etiquette were considered an elitist attempt to preserve a culture that no longer had a place in a modern egalitarian society and were counterproductive to social integration of the workplace.

No wonder the rules of etiquette were challenged, especially in the reactionary sixties and the two generations that followed. The baby boomers and that transitional generation of depression and war babies before them dispensed with the old rules and developed new codes of behavior wherever possible. They rebelled against authority in general and social conventions specifically, disdaining any authoritative edict on how to dress, act, or carry on relationships. If a particular behavior wasn't against the law, and sometimes even if it was, individuals or groups would do it.

In the past fifty years, we have seen an increase and an increasing tolerance of public incivility, rude, and inconsiderate behavior. There is a general perception that our society has lost its manners, and that short of inviting a court appearance, we take delight in flaunting behavioral norms or watching those who do. In a nationwide study entitled *Aggravating Circumstances: A Status Report on Rudeness in America* prepared for the Pew Charitable Trust by the non-profit organization Public Agenda, the majority of Americans surveyed believed rudeness is on the rise in our society and surprisingly, almost half admitted to being part of the problem. Seventy-nine percent believed lack of respect and courtesy is a serious national problem and 73 percent believed Americans treated one another with more respect in the past.[1]

Aggressive drivers, parents at youth sporting events, flagrant littering, cell phone users in public spaces, rude face-to-face attendants in retail stores, even ruder telephone customer service operators, were all mentioned by respondents in the survey and are daily anonymous irritants. It seems everyone has a story to tell about the shopper with the full basket in the quick checkout line, a healthy individual using a disabled parking spot, or the young, athletic office worker sitting in front of the granny standing in the bus aisle.

Examples of bad behavior are easy to find. Just consider celebrities like Jerry Springer, Howard Stern, Don Imus, and Maury Povich. All have made careers by celebrating rudeness. Dependent on shock for entertainment, when the shocking is commonplace, they create new frontiers of public incivility. Reality shows like *Survivor* and *The Amazing Race* reward rudeness. Rude behavior became such a problem in New York City that Mayor Giuliani, noted for his own brusque behavior, and at times prickly demeanor, made public displays of civility an initiative of his second term. Even our elected representatives, who should provide us with models of civility, have acted inappropriately at times.

Former Georgia Representative Cynthia McKinney struck a Capitol police officer when he failed to recognize her and stopped her at a checkpoint. Former Republican House Majority Leader Tom DeLay and Rep. David Obey (D-Wisconsin) got into a shoving match on the floor of the House of Representatives in 1997, and in 2006 Rep. Obey was seen on YouTube calling some of his fellow Democrats "idiot liberals."

If a list of rules of etiquette is outdated, civility is still pertinent. A voiced thank-you for a favor is not just a thank-you; it is an acknowledgment of a good deed or favor performed, and perhaps selfishly, an invitation to a repeat performance. Listening and responding in a dialogue is not just a way of showing the person with whom we are engaged that we care about them and what they are saying, it's a critical tool for the effective exchange of ideas.

Unfortunately, the medical profession is not immune to the nihilism of manners in general society. In her book, *Miss Manners Rescues Civilization,* Judith Martin devotes four pages to the healthcare profession.[2] She lists specific examples of rude behavior: systematically making patients wait for appointments, failure to treat patients with respect, skipping introductions, not asking for permission before touching a patient, not explaining procedures adequately, and discussing a patient around non-medical personnel. She devotes an entire paragraph on the manner of dress and lack of neatness of the medical profession.

The behavior of the medical community has changed, but not all of the changes are unwelcome. Following World War II, large numbers of veterans from all social strata determined to enter every profession. Many sought careers in medicine, and medical schools opened their doors to qualified applicants who might have previously been denied entrance due to class, ethnicity, or income. Initially barriers broke down slowly. Then in the general upheaval of the sixties and seventies—with the confluence of the civil rights and anti-war movements, and the push for female equality—the young, brash, bright, and self-confident men and women of that generation, found many of the rules of behavior either incomprehensible or irrational. This included a shirt and tie dress code, how long to wait for the often tardy professor before starting rounds, withholding opinions unless specifically asked, the formality of address, and standing at military attention at the bedside. They simply refused to go along. Interns discarded uniforms of all white shirts, pants, and shoes for informal dress, and scrub clothes became the new uniform of the day for rounds. Even the title of intern was discarded.

These symbolic changes reflected greater shifts in the profession itself. As the need for doctors increased, and in response to federal and state funding of care for the elderly and indigent (Medicare and Medicaid), medical school class size expanded, per capita grants to training programs were increased, and access to medical care improved. Medicine had always attracted the intellectual and the empathetic, the problem solver who wants to help a neighbor. Now the qualified student had the opportunity to enroll in medical school without regard to social class or background.

With passage of the Hart-Celler Act in 1965, legislation of The Great Society that ameliorated the restrictive immigration laws of the 1920s, foreign medical graduates, raised in alien cultures and unfamiliar with the formalities of American life, entered practice as did first generation Americans raised in ethnic communities. This resulted in a melding of cultures and behavioral norms. This social fluidity further encouraged a relaxation of arbitrary rules of conduct that served no utilitarian purpose. It's tough to define and enforce a training program dress code, already unpopular, when the Sikh surgeon wears a turban, and the Indian resident dresses in her sari for rounds. It's also discriminatory and unproductive.

As medical school classes increased so did the enrollment of women, who now make up slightly less than 50 percent of medical school students.[3] Like it or not, this has introduced gender politics into medicine. Deference in social mannerisms within the workplace—once considered courtly—is now looked upon as antiquated at best and demeaning by some. The traditional male/female, doctor/nurse hierarchical relationship has shifted as women and men assume roles in both categories. Nurses, once considered subservient to doctors, now provide first responder care in emergencies, and are included in decision making at the bedside.

Practices some might consider symbolic of respectful behavior disappeared along with the superfluous. Attending physicians arrive on the floor in jeans and with unruly facial hair. The same scrub clothes worn in the operating room and the procedure room are worn in the office, often not covered by a white coat. Doctors and nurses in the hospital, barely acquaintances, address each other on a first-name basis. Trainees and professors address each other informally. Patients are referred to as the gall bladder in room 350, or the gomer in bed six, and are addressed informally by first name, when their names are used at all. Teaching rounds are conducted without introductions, trainees eat in front of the patients—we have seen a hungry resident take the toast off a confused patient's breakfast tray during teaching rounds—and students are taught, by observation and experience, how to demean, harass, and exploit colleagues of lesser experience.

Where does the young doctor-in-training learn manners and other social skills? Medical school courses are challenged to incorporate into the curriculum an ever-enlarging body of medical science in a limited amount of time. Since all medical school students have received a college education and degree, those accepted for admissions are expected to be caring and empathetic individuals for whom training and instruction in common courtesy and good manners are not necessary. Seventeen years of elementary and high school followed by college classes in history, philosophy, and the humanities should render even the most contrary of individuals socially competent. Based on our experience with medical students, we have noted most to be exceptionally well mannered, very caring, and empathetic when they enter medical school but changed by their experiences as they train and mature.

How does this happen? For the entering students—mostly young, inexperienced, and sheltered by family and the university—life's existential problems, if considered at all, have been studied at a distance rather than experienced. When they confront death or suffering in infants and children, or a young mother or father, or watch a family grieve as they themselves feel frustrated in their attempts to alter an inevitable course, the caregiver suffers personal emotional pain, depression, and feelings of inadequacy. The defensive response of some students may be to devalue the patient and family, or trivialize the dilemma with humor and lose perspective and respect for the individuals involved. Young students, responsible for their patients' survival, exposed perhaps for the first time in their lives to the reality and absurdity of life, death, and disease, use dark, degrading humor as a temporary crutch. This can show up as inappropriate behavior and sometimes shape lifelong attitudes.

A great deal of medical education and almost all post-graduate medical instruction is mentored training. The student or newly minted doctor learns not only diagnosis, treatment, procedures, and policies from his mentors, but also social skills. Young doctors obtain their professional manners at the bedside from their senior residents in an unstructured manner and with little or no feedback from the senior physicians or patients. The senior attending physicians or professors are present to serve as role models. But today's professors are often laboratory scientists and not experienced clinicians. They may lack the interpersonal skills required to handle difficult situations. Further, the patient interactions students observe are mostly limited to highly structured and formalized rounds that rarely mimic the true environment in the hospital or the office. Contact with most patients is brief and episodic with no opportunity to observe the impact of bedside behavior on the patient or family.

When it comes to manners, medical students and residents seem to suffer from arrested development, and if students are supposed to learn behavior by example, then the system is doomed. In 1994, the *Journal of the American Medical Association* published a report "Disputes between Medical Supervisors and Trainees," citing several studies documenting misconduct and mistreatment of trainees by their supervisors and suggesting abuse and mistreatment of all kinds from a variety of sources— residents, nurses, medical students, and patients.[4] The perception is, when abuse arises, the victims have less authority than the victimizers. In one study, abuse ranged from threats of academic punishment, trivial duties assigned to punish the student, verbal abuse, belittlement, humiliation, and even threats of physical harm. Sixty-three percent of trainees reported being belittled or humiliated by more senior colleagues and over half of female trainees reported having been sexually harassed at least once, with about half the incidents arising in medical school and half during residency. The manners students learn are the manners they observe.

Medical Manners—How Times Have Changed

The history of medical etiquette is intrinsically bound with the history of medicine. Before the advent of scientific medicine, good bedside manners were often the only comfort a doctor could provide to his patient. In the ancient Greek and Roman world, manners, aesthetics, and decorum were bound to ethical values. Hippocratic teachings as in *De Medico* and *De Decenti Habitu* describe the ideal physician with explicit rules for external appearance and proper demeanor.[5]

The earliest statement of an aesthetic and ethic text is the Hippocratic Oath attributed to Hippocrates of Cos (450–370 BCE). This text consists of four elements: a preamble calling on the gods to bear witness in the swearing of the oath; a covenant describing the duties of the practitioner to the profession; a code committing the physician to certain responsibilities for the patient; and a statement in which the physician affirms the commitment to upholding the oath.[6]

The code instructs the physician in acceptable treatments for the patient such as applying dietetic measures for the benefit of the sick and to never give a deadly drug for any reason even when the patient requests one. The code also defines acceptable conduct. The physician is advised to be interested only in the benefit of the sick and to refrain from intentional injustice, mischief, and in particular sexual relations with patients.

Western medical practice and tradition changed very little with the Christianization of Europe through the Medieval and Renaissance periods. The Hippocratic Oath was adopted by Christian philosophers, who endorsed its message of the sanctity of human life and added to it the Christian principles of charity. In the early Renaissance, the concepts of ethics and aesthetics began to diverge. The role of behavior and manners changed from achieving a just, moral goal to achieving certain personal goals. The art of decorum was characterized by egotism and social calculation. Good manners were observed to improve an individual's standing in the community, not to make the world a better place to live.

Modern concepts of medical manners and bedside behavior begin with John Gregory's book *Lectures on the Duties and Qualifications of a Physician* in 1772. Gregory defines humanity as "that sensibility of heart which makes us feel for the distresses of our fellow creatures, and which of consequence incites us in the most powerful manner to relieve...Sympathy naturally engages the affection and confidence of a patient, which, in many cases, is of the utmost consequence to his recovery."[7]

Gregory's concept of manners is not about a paternalistic, self-serving manner to promote the personal interests of the physician. It is about the well-being of the patient. The dress and decorum are to gain the patient's confidence. This central interest in the well-being of the patient places the "gentleness of manner" on the same level as humanity.

In 1803, Sir Thomas Percival, a student of John Gregory, wrote *Medical Ethics*, a guide for physician behavior toward colleagues and patients. This was the result of physician misbehavior at the Royal Infirmary in Manchester, England.[8] The American Medical Association adopted a code of ethics based on Percival's guidelines at their first official meeting in Philadelphia in 1847. This code formed a contract between the profession, its patients, and the public. In return for the right to set licensing standards and educational levels, the profession, among other issues, dedicated its members to the needs of the sick. Included in the code were the Hippocratic principles, as well as rules of consultation and etiquette.[9] The code has undergone multiple revisions since then and, as revised in June 2001, is a set of nine principles, the first of which is: "A physician shall be dedicated to providing competent medical care, with compassion and **respect for human dignity and rights**" [emphasis ours].[10]

Prior to the twentieth century, formal educational requirements for physicians did not exist. Many medical schools did not require a high school education, there were no licensing or competency exams, and a student only had to pay tuition to receive a diploma. The public did not hold doctors in high esteem.

A far-reaching reform of medical education from proprietary schools to university-affiliated graduate degree programs followed publication of the *Flexner Report* in the early part of the twentieth century.[11] More and more doctors were highly educated professionals, and as medical science improved and increased their ability to care for the sick, the profession attracted the best and the brightest students. In the mid-twentieth century, the discovery of antibiotics, insulin, modern anesthesia, antiseptic surgery, and other extraordinary scientific advances further improved the perception of doctors by the general public. Medicine ranked among the most admired and respected professions and doctors were viewed in the popular media as individuals working to improve the quality and length of lives.

Popular opinion reflects conditions as they are perceived and is never static. By the twenty-first century, doctors had fallen from grace despite remarkable and innovative therapeutic advances. The portrayal of doctors on TV and in the movies documents this change and perhaps reveals at least one precipitating factor. The kind and empathetic twentieth-century doctor portrayed by Robert Young as Dr. Marcus Welby, the heroic Dr. Sam Abelman played by Paul Muni in *The Last Angry Man*, and Cary Grant's suave and gallant Dr. Noah Praetorius in the movie *People Will Talk*, displayed impeccable manners and complete devotion to the welfare of their patients. The current cast of media medicos presents a stark contrast. It includes the sarcastic, rude, and unkempt Dr. Gregory House, a doctor who abuses prescription drugs, Dr. John Dorian of *Scrubs* who has erotic daydreams while on patient rounds, and Dr. Meredith Grey of *Grey's Anatomy* whose romantic interests seem to take precedence over patient care. The odd contradiction is in older movies, the best clinicians were also the best-mannered doctors; now, the worst offenders of civil behavior are made out to be the most effective physicians.

Seventy years have elapsed between *People Will Talk* and *House*. The physician we see on the screen is no longer the preeminent, intelligent, self-assured healer with impeccable manners, and a model of behavior. In our world, the doctor is portrayed as an abrasive, self-centered, arrogant, rude, cold, and unfeeling physician.

These portrayals are far from realistic, but in some cases the caricature reveals some small truth.

Whose Manners Are These?

Boorish behavior by medical professionals is not just about generational attitudes. Consider Dr. Jesse James, a superbly trained urologist, a graduate of an Ivy League college and medical school and the recipient of training at outstanding residency programs. Dr. James is known on the surgical wards for his abrupt demeanor and often disruptive behavior. He is condescending at best and very often rude to the nurses caring for his hospitalized patients. He seems to especially enjoy berating the nurses at his patients' bedside. Dr. James mistakenly believes his behavior ensures the best and most meticulous care for his patients. However, because nurses do not enjoy caring for his patients, when nursing assignments are made, his patients are assigned to the nurse with least seniority or whoever draws the short straw. Nurses avoid him. When he rounds on his patients, the nurses make themselves scarce. Dr. James jeopardizes patient care with his outwardly rude behavior and the nurses compound the problem with passive-aggressive avoidance.

Dr. James is not likely to endear himself to those around him. If communication is poor among the health care team, even the most skillful physician will have difficulty achieving the desired results. His behavior and the effect on his colleagues negatively affect the health of his patients.

Dr. James's behavior reflects ignorance in social skills. He suffers from a lack of training in bedside manners. Unfortunately, his patients and colleagues must suffer as well. As we have pointed out, medical schools pay little to no attention to training students in courtesy and manners or building skills in social behavior. The assumption is that the desire to do good necessarily leads to proper behavior. This assumption is as common in medicine as it is in everyday affairs. As Judith Martin writes, the error is "that from personal virtue, acceptable social behavior will follow effortlessly. All you need is a good heart, and the rest will take care of itself."[12]

Not so. We have noted a remarkable change and a lack of consensus in what is considered acceptable behavior. While we do not object to the trend toward an easing of formality, the corresponding decrease in civility, from the trivial omission of a title of address to the critical display of disrespect inherent in any public confrontation, has affected the quality of patient care.

Informality does not have to be tied to rude behavior. Along with relaxed standards of personal dress and the move away from plush office design, with which we have no complaint and even welcome, we have seen a laxness in neat appearance and personal hygiene. We have observed some offices, hospital rooms, and corridors in serious need of a cleanup crew. An open shirt collar looks so much nicer when connected to a cleaned and pressed shirt. Facial hair can be neatly groomed, long tresses washed and combed.

Despite the loosening of formality in greetings between peers and colleagues, it is still not proper for doctors and nurses to address patients more than three times their age by first names upon initial meetings, or ever without permission. These may seem like trivial concerns, but they illustrate the bigger issue: the dignity of the patient and the need to address patients with empathy and politeness. Ignore those qualities and there can be no hope for open communication, and it is open communication that is critical to the doctor's improved understanding of your complaint. Open communication also means you will have a better understanding of your treatment and promotes mutual trust. Civility provides a basis for professional behavior that encourages positive, beneficial human interaction.

Modern medical care is all about teamwork. Individual members of the team must support and respect each other. Saving a life is like flying to the moon; it takes a lot of individuals each working in concert with the other. When physicians, office, or hospital employees are rude or disrespectful, they will be avoided and their patients will suffer poorly coordinated care.

Your Doctors' Manners Matter

Do Good Manners Need Guidelines?

Isn't it enough for the doctor to be pure of heart and want to do the right thing? Even in everyday personal exchanges, without guidelines for best behavior we would not know what to expect when approaching another, and have no way to measure rude behavior. Taking offense if poorly treated would be considered inappropriate because there would be no rules as to what is poor treatment and what is fair treatment. Anarchy of manners would follow, and any behavior would be acceptable up to the point where the law is broken.

Imagine how this might work in a medical clinic. The internist decides his patients should sit naked in the exam room, reasoning that it will save time and the patient can dress when the visit is over. The surgeon calls his patients at home with their lab results after ten p.m. He wants to be sure to connect with them. The psychiatrist schedules all his morning patients to arrive in his waiting room at nine a.m. and the afternoon patients by two p.m. If he has a no-show, he can call a patient on his waiting list to fill in the empty slot. Sure the patient with the noon and five p.m. slot will wait three hours, but the psychiatrist is likely to maintain a full schedule.

Of course these examples are ridiculous (and actual examples), but so is a lunch-stained lab coat or not explaining to a patient why they need certain tests or medications. We expect a certain amount of privacy, neatness, and order in our doctors' offices. Although there are no laws* addressing office management, there cannot be any argument about "clothing the naked" being both moral behavior and good manners, and alleviating anxiety a mark of the compassionate person.

Rules of behavior do change and are reflective of society, but moral principles such as consideration, respect, and tolerance do not. Rapid changes in medical science affects our system of delivering medical care; technology revolutionizes how we communicate both in the medical community and in general society. Acceptable behavior, once thought as established as arithmetic, now seems to need redefinition with every election cycle. Quality medical care based on good manners reflects those unchanging moral principles.

---

* With the exception of breaches of confidentiality. The Health Insurance Portability and Accountability Act (HIPAA) made it illegal to share patient information without the patient's consent.

Your Doctors' Manners Matter

Chapter One
Manners, Medicine, and Morals
Issues Addressed in this Chapter

- Doctors with good manners are more likely to listen closely to their patients and encourage their patients to tell the complete story about what is troubling them. This makes for improved medical care.

- When your doctor treats you with respect, you are more likely to follow the doctor's advice.

- Every society has rules of social behavior; acceptable behavior in the medical office has changed over the years.

- Doctors communicate the principles of medical ethics through courteous behavior.

- Moral principles such as consideration, respect, and tolerance do not change. Quality medical care based on good manners reflects unchanging moral principles.

- In many areas, doctors no longer enjoy the high esteem they once did. This is at least in part due to a change in the way doctors relate to their patients.

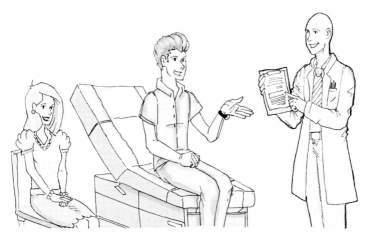

Chapter Two

Compassion and Communication

The practice of medicine is an art, not a trade; a calling, not a business; a calling in which your heart will be exercised equally with your head.

— William Osler, 1849–1919

People take cues from the institutions around them. In a major emergency department in our city—25,000 square feet of spotless, shining, tiled and glass-walled cubicles—every hallway displays the sign "Courtesy & Respect." Yet patients are left waiting for hours before being seen, and other patients wait for what seems forever to be admitted to as yet unassigned rooms while their anxious families mark time in the waiting area unaware of the fate of their loved ones.

Maybe the hospital is understaffed or overcrowded, but it takes just a few seconds for the nurse or ward clerk to visit and reassure the patient they have not been forgotten, or to keep anxiously waiting families informed of the patient's progress. Why should the hospital or your doctor's office behave differently from a restaurant where the diners are warned if they have to wait for a table or are notified if their meal is delayed? Even the airlines have learned how important it is to keep the traveler notified of a delay and inform them of the cause. We expect common courtesy and good manners in business dealings. There is no good reason to settle for less in our medical care.

Doctors and nurses work with patients at a most vulnerable period in their lives, during an illness, when listening attentively to the patient and encouraging questions is critical to providing good care. Yet not a day passes when a patient, family member, nurse, therapist, or physician does not take offense or feel bruised by the callous, inattentive, or disagreeable behavior of a colleague or coworker.

Organized medicine recognizes the importance of respect for human rights and the dignity of the patient when providing care. The first of the AMA "Principles of Ethics" requires physicians to respect human dignity and rights. The four commonly held principles of bioethics acknowledge that every person has human dignity and must be treated with and is entitled to respect.† Recognizing the principle of human dignity, the unique quality each of us possesses as humans, is essential in working through bioethical issues. The doctor who demonstrates concern and treats patients with respect marks the compassionate caregiver.

You want your doctor to respect his or her patients. It's likely you want your doctor to respect all humanity. If the doctor's actions in your encounter lead you to suspect the opposite, you might wonder about the commitment to your health. In any event, you might view any opinion as to diagnosis and treatment as suspect, even self-serving, and you will probably not heed any instructions received or return to the office for follow-up.

Of course not every disagreeable encounter with a doctor or nurse is an indication of depravity, just as not every individual display of good manners is an indication of a person's essential morality. Ruthless dictators and sociopathic financial manipulators may

---

† These principles are widely used when making decisions about medical ethics and are based on the idea that human dignity requires respect. These four principles are patient autonomy, nonmaleficence, (the doctor never intentionally creates a needless harm or injury to the patient), beneficence (the doctor provides some benefit to the patient), and the principle of fairness in the allocation of resources.

display impeccable manners. But what are we to think when the doctor who just entered the room does not have the courtesy to introduce himself or state his role, or the nurse or technician who wakes us to change the bed linen does not murmur an apology?

Attention to good manners is particularly important in the hospital and medical office where many barriers of social convention are altered: unilateral nakedness, conversations about ailments, intrusive questioning, all banned in civil company, are critical to the medical encounter. So with these barriers dispensed with voluntarily, it is especially important that the doctor and staff act in accordance with other conventions of respectful behavior—uninterrupted listening, solicitous attention to physical comfort, agreeable demeanor, and pleasant surroundings. You get your impression of a doctor's capability, not from the physician's medical expertise—few patients have the training to make that evaluation—but rather from the doctor's concern for you as a patient and a human being. That concern is conveyed through manners, a willingness to consider your feelings, preferences, and views, and an ability to communicate with you.

The famous Johns Hopkins physician Philip Tumulty addressed the issue of communicating with patients in his 1970 address to third year medical students:

Your Doctors' Manners Matter

Actually, what many patients miss and resent today is the inability to communicate with their physician in a meaningful manner. Patients have questions they want answered, fears requiring dissipation, misunderstandings that need clarification and abysmal ignorance about themselves that demands enlightenment. Today, many patients with serious health problems leave their physician's offices with less comprehension of what is wrong and what they must do to get well than the average customer understands about his car when he drives it out of his repair shop. And if the patient feels deprived of adequate communication with his physician, family members are totally devoid of it. No wonder the resentment.[1]

How well you are treated as a patient in the medical office or in the hospital is not just a matter of attitude. It is a moral and ethical concern. Professor Cheshire Calhoun of Arizona State University, writing in the journal *Philosophy and Public Affairs*, includes civility as a moral virtue whose function is to communicate basic moral attitudes.[2] Professor Calhoun makes the point that the importance of civility is in the *"display* [author emphasis] of respect, tolerance, and considerateness…" Judith Martin, in her book, describes manners as the "modest partner" of morality, and that in order to avoid being offensive, we must treat each other with respect.[3]

Rude and uncivil behavior is often either ignored or given a pass. This leads to an escalation of misbehavior and a tolerance to tactlessness. Take for example Hank Johnson, a conscientious physician who always goes the extra mile for his patients. In addition to serving on numerous hospital committees, he also serves as a lay preacher in his church. One morning he was overheard criticizing the nursing supervisor, Susan Butler, who was responsible for the area where his patient had been admitted. Miss Butler is an experienced and respected nurse, highly skilled and capable, and known for her ability to defuse difficult situations. Apparently Dr. Johnson's patient had not been weighed despite orders to do so. In view and hearing of others, the doctor lost no opportunity to inform Nurse Butler of his poor opinion of the care his patient was receiving, and moved on to a general critique of her crew. Their voices were not raised, but his words and demeanor clearly indicated his displeasure. She nodded and apologized and tried to appease him with an explanation. After a few minutes, he walked off the floor, frowning and shaking his head. After the incident Susan was asked why Hank, whom she considered a valued colleague, was being so rude.

"Rude? Dr. Johnson? No. He was unhappy because he thought the nurses had ignored his order to weigh his patient. But his patient refused to be weighed. I told him it wasn't the nurse's fault."

"Did he apologize?"

"What for? He was worried about his patient. That's how he gets."

The story was related to a committee studying ways to improve professional relations, a committee Dr. Johnson serves on. No names were used, but after the meeting, Hank came up to the committee chair, a close friend of his and asked if the story was about him. Told it was, he looked abashed. "I didn't realize I behaved like that," he said. "I should have apologized."

This story illustrates the crux of the problem. Uncivil and often rude physician behavior in the professional setting is often accepted, tolerated, and excused. The perpetrator is never called out. The doctor who believes aggressive behavior is an effective management tool is not made aware of the effect of the behavior on colleagues and is surprised and insulted when feelings are hurt and blame is given.

You expect excellent medical care, your doctor expects his colleagues to treat him or her in a respectful fashion, and the nurses and allied healthcare personnel expect every member of the team to be respectful and supportive. When all involved in the healthcare team are familiar with the manners expected of them, incidents of misunderstanding and hurt feelings will be reduced, and perceptions of rude and uncaring behavior will be minimized or even eliminated.

It is not likely that enforcing rules of etiquette, often non-utilitarian, will encourage the virtues of compassion and respect, or stimulate intellectual curiosity. Dress codes do not make an effective staff, although sloppy dress can result in perceptions of inferior care. Formal address does not equate with empathy, although artificial familiarity can offend. Polite behavior is not a complete indicator of a physician's ability, although as we have argued, it is one of the most visible ways you can assess a physician's respect for his patients.

We recognize that most bad behavior in the medical setting arises, not out of callousness, or meanness, or expected personal gain, but rather is a result of one of two circumstances. Either the individual exhibiting the bad manners is unaware of appropriate behavior in any given situation, or emotions have run high and guidelines on how to handle a difficult interaction are lacking. Behavior one person perceives as rude another might consider appropriate to the situation.

When unsatisfactory interactions between doctors and patients and between medical professionals lead to increased tension and hurt feelings, the resulting stress requires a great deal more effort to resolve than simply improving communication. These conflicts are best avoided. A shared knowledge of what constitutes civility in interactions and common expectations of behavior can reduce conflicts and improve communication and mutual understanding. Commonly held conventions of behavior among medical professionals and between caregivers and patients will go a long way toward eliminating offensive behavior arising out of unmet expectations. Rules governing civil behavior serve to place everyone on an equal footing by knowing what to expect from each other. Judith Martin believes the "objection to 'rules' of behavior is not that we wish not to be civil, rather each of us would prefer to decide which courtesies we wish to observe and which we don't."[4]

Knowing What to Expect and How That Affects Your Medical Care

To be fair, medical institutions do take steps to educate patients on what to expect from their encounter. Hospitals and physician offices usually provide some information concerning billing details and how to resolve billing issues. Pediatric and obstetrical offices counsel young families on office hours and physician availability. On admission to the hospital, a representative counsels patients and families on the rules of the hospital ward, hands out pamphlets on procedures, and explains visiting hours, parking, and paying the bill.

On close examination, however, this is all information given for the convenience and benefit of the caregiver and not for the patient. Patients are not given information on who has access to their room, when testing will be done, how to voice preferences as to when not to be disturbed or how to be addressed. Patient rights, if mentioned at all, are limited to a pamphlet and a plaque on the wall, and the patient is expected to conform to the medical establishment's idea of how to act rather than the medical personnel conforming to norms of manners and civility.

Common courtesy requires anyone having contact with you to introduce themselves and state their role. The hospital or medical office environment is no different in this regard than any other place of commerce. Adult patients should always be addressed by their family name. Neat grooming expresses an air of respect. You should always be informed of any planned tests, their purpose, and when and how you will be notified of the results. In the hospital, you should know who will see you when you are in various states of undress, and how you can object to rounds attended by staff unfamiliar to you. Housekeeping, dietary, and lab personnel should knock and ask for permission before entering your room. There are times, it seems, as if hospitalized patients have less knowledge about their rights than prison inmates.

Your Doctors' Manners Matter

A disconnect in the behavior colleagues expect of each other can also result in problems. We understand our colleagues would rather make up their own rules and extend some considerations but not others. But we believe, as does Miss Manners, that this creates anarchy of manners. As Miss Manners writes, "People making up their own rules and deciding which courtesies they want to observe, and which they don't, is exactly the problem that has been identified as incivility and lack of consideration."[5] The doctor is clueless as to why the nurses feel he or she is condescending, sexist, rude, or demeaning. The nurses in turn do not agree with the doctor's evaluation of them as disrespectful, bossy, or uninterested.

You expect your doctor to observe at least the basic elements of civility. Absent a set of rules to govern interactions, the result can spell disaster for the patient, create an unfortunate impression about the doctor, result in large personnel turnover, and leave doctor and nurse or technician feeling abused or demeaned, angry and insulted.

In a manners-based medical office, the staff will communicate by their words and deeds that their patients are individuals deserving respect, consideration, and tolerance. Manners-based medicine in the clinic, office, and hospital improves relations among colleagues and with other healthcare workers, and we hope creates a better impression of the profession as a whole.

No other profession, with the possible exceptions of the clergy and moral philosophers, is more imbued with the concept of human dignity and worth than the medical profession. It is by our actions in our everyday lives, showing good manners, that we demonstrate the intrinsic value each of us acknowledges in the other, simply by being a healthcare worker. The healthcare profession offers special situations that elevate the usefulness of good manners from a guide for acting in an agreeable manner in everyday situations, to providing guidelines for the efficiency and coordination necessary to save life and limb in potentially chaotic situations. In the chapters to follow, you will read what behavior to expect from your doctor and what to expect in the office and the hospital.

Chapter Two
Compassion and Communication
Issues Addressed in this Chapter

- The first of the AMA "Principles of Ethics" requires physicians to respect human dignity and rights.
- The compassionate caregiver communicates well with patients and treats patients with respect.
- Acting in a civil manner communicates basic moral attitudes.
- Rude and uncivil behavior by physicians leads to a cycle of unacceptable behavior resulting in poor quality medical care.
- As a patient, you have a right to expect civility and good manners.
- If you know what to expect from a caring doctor you will choose a doctor who cares for you.

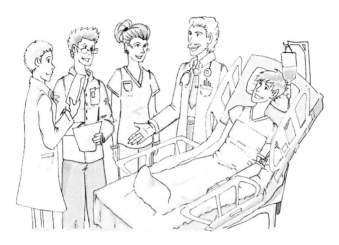

Chapter Three

Behavior of the Effective Physician

The physician's job is to treat and care for people; not to just diagnose and cure an illness.

– Cary Grant in the movie *People Will Talk*, 1951

A Doctor's Choice

How should a doctor act? What constitutes good manners in the doctor's office? Professor Sarah Buss, writing in the academic journal *Ethics* about the moral significance of manners in society, notes "one of the primary objectives of…manners is to encourage us to make ourselves *agreeable*"[1] [emphasis in original].

Professor Buss describes the most important lessons in manners as "the lessons in how to avoid being discourteous, impolite, rude, inconsiderate, offensive, insulting." To flout these lessons, she writes, is not only impolite, it is immoral. Judith Martin, writing about manners and etiquette, and Professor Sarah Buss, addressing manners and morality, agree that people have a basic moral obligation to make themselves agreeable to others.

Medical professionalism includes as one of the core values, a moral commitment to medical service based on "the potential for health and illness and on a resultant respect for the inestimable value of human life and health."[2] Speaking what Professor Buss calls the "subtle language of good manners" is how the doctor or the members of the staff say, "I respect you," and give reassurances you are worthy of respect. If a show of respect requires good manners, then good manners is not only what the patient should expect when visiting the doctor, it is a core value of good medical care.

The doctor must make it clear that you are worth treating with respect, not only to satisfy the ethical principle, but because when patients are treated with respect, they will believe the doctor cares about their welfare. Just as importantly, as Professor Buss points out, "[I]t is precisely because treating people with courtesy is a direct way of acknowledging their dignity that treating them rudely can undermine their belief in their own intrinsic worth."[3] The practice of good manners is especially important in medical care where the requirements of a thorough evaluation, if not conducted in an agreeable manner, can be stressful and embarrassing. There are few situations where a person is more vulnerable to assaults on their self-esteem than sitting in the doctor's waiting room ill, or in pain, or fearful of survival.

Manners are a way of one person communicating to another the message: I believe you have dignity, and I respect that. As Dr. Buss states, "When we treat one another politely, we are expressing respect for one another…We are, in effect, saying: 'I respect you,' 'I acknowledge your dignity.'"[4]

Good manners are not only a form of communication, good manners *foster* good communication. When you go to the doctor for a consultation, the unstated request you are making to the doctor is to work with you to improve a condition or maintain good health. A display of good manners signals that the doctor is willing to cooperate with you in that venture, that you have made a reasonable request and the doctor will devote time to fulfill it. Anything less than this response would limit the effectiveness of your consultation. Either you might not be entirely forthcoming about the history of your illness, or you might view the recommended treatments with suspicion and might not follow the plan.

Most of the time you spend with the doctor is in conversation, allowing you to tell the story of what is bothering you. If you are not comfortable and ready to talk about your problem, if you are intimidated or rushed, if you feel the doctor and the staff do not respect you as an individual, if for whatever reason you do not express your fears, your story will be incomplete. If the doctor does not hear your complete story, if you do not have the chance to communicate what you believe is bothering you, you will have less confidence in the diagnosis and prescribed treatment, and the likelihood that you will reliably follow the recommendations is reduced.

Although all medical students have heard the aphorism, "When you hear hoofbeats, don't look for zebras,"‡ it is also true that the physician has to guard against missing the uncommon disease. The ability to tell your story fully, voice your concerns, state what you believe your problem is due to, are all critical to the delivery of good medical care. An attentive doctor, listening closely, making eye contact, not interrupting, will encourage you to tell your story. The more of your story you tell, the more likely you are to give the doctor the information needed to make the correct diagnosis and provide good follow-up care. This is illustrated by the following story.

---

‡ Meaning common diseases commonly occur.

Your Doctors' Manners Matter

* * *

Mary Carruth (not her real name) first came to see Dr. Silver after an eight-month history of heart failure. Her cardiologist had diagnosed her as having hypertrophic cardiomyopathy, an unusual disease, but not a rare one, occurring in as many as 1/500 people in the general population. Some people with this condition, a thickening of the heart muscle, have no symptoms and for some it can cause fatigue and shortness of breath. This disease is the most common cause of sudden death in young athletes in the US.

The usual course of the disorder is to be stable for decades on the medication her first cardiologist recommended. Mary (she preferred her given name) had been followed closely and taken her medication, but despite this, her weakness and heart failure progressed. She had been hospitalized six times at the medical center near her North Georgia home. It was a new, large facility, just five years old and filled with state-of-the-art equipment. Her cardiologist, a well-trained, technologically competent physician, thought her worsening condition was due to her failure to follow his recommendations.

Most of Mary's contacts in the cardiologist's office were with the physician assistant, including her history and her first and most complete physical examination. Her longest conversations with the doctor followed her procedures, when he told her the results of her tests.

When she called the cardiologist's office, despite asking for the doctor on each occasion, she spoke only with the physician's assistant who advised her to continue the medication until her next visit. While her doctor ordered additional tests, his discussion of the results did not always provide Mary with information meaningful to her.

Mary had a very supportive family of six siblings, uncles and aunts, all of whom lived near her in rural North Georgia on farms they had worked for more than four generations. She was upset that her husband thought she was not so sick that she could not do her housework, and he seemed to be resentful that she was ill. He never discussed her illness with her physicians, and they never suggested he accompany her to the cardiologist's office so he could learn about her disease, its management, and her deteriorating course.

As her health declined, her family insisted their general practitioner, who they all saw on a regular basis and who had known Mary for twenty years, find another cardiologist to offer a second opinion.

Dr. Silver sat down with Mary and asked her about the course of her illness from the very beginning. She said there had been so many problems, hospital admissions, and tests she could not remember them all. With a little prompting, she told a story of progressive fatigue, no energy, feeling tired all the time. When she tried to do housework, she had to rest between rooms.

Just walking to the second level of her home was exhausting, and she had to sit on the top of the stairs to recover. She returned time and again to her cardiologist who repeated her blood studies and her electrocardiogram and echocardiogram. She remembered at least three hospitalizations where she had repeat cardiac catheterizations performed. And all this despite scrupulously following her complicated medication schedule and diet.

Mary had the pale complexion of an individual with poor heart function. While she was overweight, she was not obese. Careful observation of the veins in her neck demonstrated she had not taken on too much extra fluid, and that she was on the correct diuretic dose, always a concern in patients with heart failure. The apical impulse, where the heart beats against the chest wall just under her breast, is usually easily felt in patients with hypertrophic cardiomyopathy, yet it could not be felt at all. In addition, her heart tones were very soft, another unusual finding in patients with that condition. An unusual course of the disease despite standard treatment and unexpected physical findings led Dr. Silver to believe he was dealing with something other than the given diagnosis.

Rather than repeat her tests, he reviewed what had been done—her electrocardiogram, echocardiograms, and cardiac caths. He could see the progressive changes typical of a rare heart condition called Primary Amyloid Heart Disease.

Once he was absolutely sure of the diagnosis, he felt he could provide Mary and her family with an honest and thorough assessment of her illness. Although the prognosis was dismal, there was still much to do to make her life easier. For one thing, she no longer had to feel her illness was a result of her failure to follow the doctor's directions. For another, after educating the family about her illness, they had a better appreciation of Mary's daily struggle to carry out her activities and were eager to provide the support she needed. Mary's family doctor, a man she and her family trusted, was brought back into the loop. He received detailed reports. Dr. Silver discontinued several of her medications, some of which were harmful, the others not necessary, and together with her family and physician, he developed lifestyle changes appropriate for her condition. On a simplified but more effective treatment plan, and with a more realistic outlook for her future, her family members and friends rallied around to provide support and comfort. Her daughter, who lived away from home, moved in to help care for her.

Dr. Silver promised to provide all the care and support she and her family needed and to be available to answer any questions they had. He also promised to continue to research the literature to be sure she had the opportunity to receive any new therapies as they became available. For Mary there was no cure, but she could be helped. Knowledge of the true disease process allowed her physicians to help her and her family understand her condition and what she required.

What Mary needed was a caring and empathetic physician willing to sit down with her and believe the story she had to tell. Her family physician, who knew Mary professionally and socially for many years, could now provide her medical care since no sophisticated medical regimen was necessary.

It was important to earn Mary's trust and respect, otherwise she would be no more satisfied with Dr. Silver's exam and opinion than she was with her first cardiologist. If respect and trust are not established, then the consultation is a lost opportunity for healing. Mary lost confidence in her first cardiologist. Not just because her condition worsened, but because of his approach to her problems.

* * *

Mary's experience is far from unique. The single most striking change in medicine in the last forty years is not one of the new, incredible, and astounding technologies, but the loss of confidence patients have in their physicians. *The New York Times* reported that when doctors are arrogant, patronizing, dismissive, callous, impatient, or judgmental, patients do not trust the diagnosis that results from the consultation or follow the recommendations.

What must physicians do to earn back the trust of their patients? Dr. Tumulty, in a 1978 speech to the Johns Hopkins medical students called "The Art of Healing," had good advice for medical students. Look for these characteristics in your doctor:

> A clinician must be patient and forbearing, strong yet gentle, unselfish of his time and unstinting in his efforts. He must be willing to bite his tongue and to turn his cheek. He must have an attentive ear as well as the ability to question probingly. His attitude must create trust and confidence, and his manner thoughtfulness and security.
>
> He must hear what the patient doesn't say and be sensitive to the anguish which cannot be expressed. Patients are anxious; they are frightened; they inwardly anticipate the very worst, although they may cover up with apparent lack of concern. Some are very brave, while others cling in terror. All grasp tightly to life, and in all, some glimmer of hope, no matter how flickering, is essential to the vitality of their spirit. [5]

"Can't Get No Satisfaction"

For the first half of the last century, the social framework in organized medicine promoted cooperation, self-regulation, non-competitive behavior, and collegiality.

Your Doctors' Manners Matter

Legal and academic challenges during the era of social and economic disruption from 1960–1980 claimed that such an organized network was nothing more than a means of monopolizing trade. Together with the increasingly large economic role of the federal government through Medicare and Medicaid grants—plus anti-trust litigation against doctor groups and the influence of managed care organizations driven at least in part by the profit incentive—the ethic of collegiality and civility, while not eliminated, seemed to take a back seat to competition. Many healthcare organizations, responding to the government and the business community, especially healthcare insurers, adopted business models that gave increasing importance to a profitable bottom line.[§]

The change in behavior among and between doctors and between doctors and administrators of medical institutions, whether by coincidence or as a result of pressures to behave in a more business oriented way, affects the way you are seen and treated as a patient. In the worst organizations, patients are dehumanized and become a commodity. On more than one occasion, we have heard patients referred to as "job security."

But the pendulum swings both ways. We doubt if poor manners are a result of a deficiency in medical professionalism. Most of the colleagues and staff we have

---

[§] The hope was that market forces would lower the cost of care. Not working out too well.

met in our nearly a century of combined practices are well motivated and truly concerned about their patients. Doctors who act in a disrespectful manner are either not knowledgeable about what patients expect, or are not aware of the messages sent by their actions or the actions of their office staff. It is therefore important for the doctor and staff to "act the language," to behave in such a way that you understand they care about your health. Recognizing the changes in the way patients are being treated, organized medical education has instituted required curriculum in medical schools to teach medical professionalism to student doctors and residents in training. Training in good manners can be part of that curriculum.

You will feel satisfied with your visit to the doctor's office if, upon leaving, you feel confident in your doctor's abilities and trust that any recommended testing and treatment are in your best interests. Likewise, the doctor will consider the visit successful if you understand and agree with the recommendations. This is an indication of your trust and confidence in the doctor's conclusions, and here is where a problem exists.

On what do you base your trust? You can't reasonably be expected to perform an evaluation of your doctor's abilities, knowledge, or training. Other than the recommendations given by friends (who may have one or two experiences with the doctor; very little to go on) or other physicians' recommendations, the average visitor to the doctor has little information to evaluate the quality of care they receive. You inspect the diplomas hung on the wall. You are supposed to be impressed by the pictures of civic leaders and celebrities with whom the doctor is shaking hands and who are presumably his patients. You read the certificates from organizations with important sounding names. But the most important impression is the one you form based on the way the doctor acts. His bedside manner.

You may not be able to evaluate your doctor's surgical technique, but you do know what it is to be agreeable, and when you enter the doctor's office, you have some expectations that the reception you will be given and the treatment you will receive will be so. Chances are you are willing to give the doctor a degree of slack for the state of the office surroundings, although as we will discuss later, the physical environment can say a lot about the practice. You will probably also accept a waiting time if it is not interminable. But you expect the office staff to treat you politely and in a civil way, and when it comes to the doctor, the person to whom we literally and figuratively bare ourselves, we expect a standard of behavior that is higher than what we expect from others.

One Physician's Opinion

In 2006, George Beller, a past president of the American College of Cardiology, wrote the following in an editorial in the *Journal of the American College of Cardiology*. His wife was suffering from a serious illness, and he made the following recommendations related to the behavior of the doctors responsible for her care:

> The patient should expect the physician to be caring and empathetic, take the time to explain what was found in the medical evaluation, describe the disease process in lay terms, not hurry the patient when answering questions, show sensitivity and compassion when having to relate bad news, display a realistic but positive attitude about treatment plans, and fully explain why certain tests are being ordered and specific drugs or procedures are being recommended.[6]

This is how the doctor earns your trust. Dr. David Pendleton and co-authors, in the book *The New Consultation: Developing Doctor-Patient Communication*, identified the following five key issues a doctor should address for a consultation to be effective.[7] [By effective, the authors mean the consultation results in an improvement in your health.]

The doctor must:
(a) understand the problem,
(b) understand the patient,

(c) the doctor and the patient must agree on the problem,
(d) share decisions and responsibility,
(e) and maintain a relationship.

Over the course of an effective consultation, you will develop a firm understanding of what to do to improve your health and why, and your resolve and commitment to follow the doctor's recommendations will strengthen.

Keeping in mind that practical considerations do limit the amount of time the doctor can spend with each patient, at the end of the consultation you should leave the office satisfied that you have been encouraged to tell your story, that the doctor listened attentively and understood what you said, and that you understand what further tests and treatments are to be done and why. It is important that you, as the patient, are in full agreement with the follow-up plan. Although the doctor may be the expert in charge of the consultation, when you leave the office, you are in charge of your care. You must believe and understand the diagnosis and the plan to be able to effectively execute it.

Ninety percent of diagnoses can be made by listening carefully to a skillfully elicited history, yet Howard Beckman, MD, and colleagues have shown that on the average, the patient gets interrupted by the doctor's questioning within the first twenty-three seconds of telling their story.[8] If you are unable to completely tell your story, you might not have confidence that the doctor came to the correct conclusions about your illness.

Listening is important, but not only listening improves your trust in the doctor. A number of studies on physician-patient communication demonstrate that health outcomes are improved by verbal and non-verbal behaviors. How a physician dresses, facial expressions, how you are approached, and whether your physician's attention is focused on you all play important roles in building your trust in the doctor and how likely you are to follow the advice you receive.

In his popular book *How Doctors Think*, Harvard physician Dr. Jerome Groopman notes that freedom of patient speech is necessary for the doctor to reach a correct diagnosis and therapeutic plan.[9] Referencing other researchers, he notes how the interview process not only exchanges information between patient and doctor and doctor and patient, but also establishes trust and "a sense of mutual liking." It's the "liking" part, based on mutual respect, that results in improved patient follow-up, what doctor's call compliance, or adherence to the therapeutic plan.

Looking back to Mary C.'s story, she did not receive the correct diagnosis and an appropriate treatment plan until she had the opportunity to sit down with her new doctor and tell her complete story. The heartache and suffering Mary experienced was a personal loss, but the wasted doctor's visits, unneeded and extremely expensive procedures, and excess medication are added costs, not just to Mary but to all healthcare consumers.

It's Not Me, It's the Machine

Some of the negative views patients have of their doctors are due to a failure by the doctor to establish a relationship, and some are due to an estrangement of doctor and patient due to the depersonalization of medical care. You give your medical history online, before you even get to the office. On arrival to the office, you are again asked the questions you answered in your questionnaire, and now you start to wonder why you bothered. When you do finally get to tell your story to the doctor, usually in response to a variation of the question "What brought you here today," the doctor is sitting at a desk facing a computer and typing your responses into a form.

Once in the exam room, many doctors no longer ask their patients to disrobe, instead listening to the chest and feeling the abdomen over clothes. When we were students, an exam like that would have resulted in dismissal from the clinic. Lewis Thomas, a respected researcher from the Rockefeller University, now deceased, wrote many essays and editorials in the *New England Journal of Medicine*. He noted that "medicine is no longer the laying on of hands; it is more like the reading of signals from machines."[10] CT scans, PET scans, MRIs, and ultrasounds have replaced probing fingers and stethoscopes.

The physician, once the valued confidant and adviser for the family who assisted not only with the medical problems, but also with the social and emotional ones, is no longer in practice. Today's doctors are working just as hard, and putting in the long hours, but in a vastly different medical environment complicated by the demands of managed care, profit-oriented medical management companies, health maintenance organizations, and the need for increasingly focused specialty practices. Practices are not only divided by organs or disease types, such as neurology or endocrinology or cardiac surgery, but also by the location where the patients are seen: Emergency department doctors, hospitalists, health maintenance clinic doctors, multispecialty group practices. All this compartmentalization makes an ongoing relationship with one physician more difficult and seem less and less important.

What has been lost in the rush to technology is the trust that is established by face-to-face time with the doctor and a sharing of secrets we are hesitant to share with even our closest friends. Lost is the gentle, yet expert, physical exam where probing fingers identify and even reproduce an area of discomfort or pain, followed by a sympathetic response by the doctor. If a lump in the belly is carefully identified and circumscribed by the doctor's palpation, our confidence in the examiner is established. If the doctor takes the time to listen carefully to the chest, elicit the wheeze we had the evening before, or has the stethoscope over our heart when it breaks out of normal rhythm, we are confident the doctor will figure out our problem. If questions elicit the symptoms we forgot to mention, an indication the doctor is on the right track, or when the sympathetic nod acknowledges our fears and presumptions, we know our concerns will be addressed.

Bernard Lown, the famous Boston cardiologist, clinician, and Nobel Prize winner, expressed this opinion in his 1996 memoir *The Lost Art of Healing*: "The American public is suspicious, distrustful of, even antagonistic to, the profession."[11] He comments that a doctor establishes credentials as a caring practitioner by listening attentively, and he sees the trust between patient and doctor, established over several millennia, slipping away. This lack of trust is not only a problem for the individual practitioner and the patient, the problem extends to the role organized medicine will play in the ongoing reinvention of the medical care system in America. Medicine as a profession needs to re-establish its position as a trusted adviser and steward of the patient's health, an invaluable partner in care and an indispensable resource for the health of the community and the nation.

One opinion that has surfaced in our country's debate about the best way to finance our medical care is that a trusting personal relationship with our doctors is missing. We take pride in believing we have the best medical care in the world even as our statistics for infant mortality, heart disease, patient satisfaction, life expectancy, and medical errors demonstrate otherwise. Newspaper articles air complaints about arrogant and difficult physicians, patients complain about missed diagnoses, inability to get appointments due to inadequate insurance policies, and doctors opting out of government programs that insure older patients or patients living near or below the poverty line.

Life-saving advances in medicine improve our health, and in the end, better health is what we want. Today's doctors know more about diseases, have more and better diagnostic tests and treatment options than ever before, and can help more patients regain well-being than any previous generation of physicians. Indeed, for most patients their first priority when choosing a physician or surgeon is knowledge and skill. Yet many patients leave the physician's office dissatisfied and unconvinced. They believe their health is not the doctor's first concern. It is useless to diagnose an illness and recommend a course of testing and treatment if you do not trust in the doctor's opinion. Even if an uncomplicated illness can be rapidly diagnosed with little patient history, and most can, and all that is needed to confirm the diagnosis is an abbreviated physical exam, the respect and trust that should develop between you and the doctor during the office visit can make the difference in how determined you will be to follow up with diagnostic studies and treatment plans. When the longest conversation you have is with the billing office, if you never really get to know who is in charge of your medical care, the likelihood that you will closely follow your physician's advice is diminished and the outcome of the consultation will be less than satisfactory.

There are many reasons patient-doctor communication can break down. In fairness, the busy, overworked physician who has just administered to a terminally ill patient might appear brusque to a patient with a cold and not remember there are no trivial complaints. Each patient's complaints are important to them. If you feel the doctor is distracted, do not hesitate to speak up. Try a statement like "Doctor, I am not sure you understand how ill I really feel." Or you may be in a heightened emotional state and not listening to or understanding what your doctor is saying. The anxiety about your illness can cause so much discomfort you just want out of the doctor's office away from the source of your unease about your illness and your mortality. It is for this reason it's a good idea to have a family member or a friend accompany you to the doctor.

If you find you are asking the same question over and over, in the same words, the reason may be the doctor has not made the answers clear enough, or perhaps you are asking one question, but really want the answer to another and are afraid to ask it. Try to rephrase the question. One of the goals of the consultation is to discover and resolve your fears. This may reveal the true concern.

Professor Cheshire Calhoun writes in the essay "Expecting Common Decency" that the helping professions, medicine, nursing, and teaching, among others, "take on a special responsibility for promoting something of moral value that those outside the profession do not have a similar responsibility to promote."[12] For doctors, this means behavior that exhibits caring, empathy, expertise, compassion, and a commitment to medical service.

Setting an example is not the main means of influencing another, it is the only means.
   – **Albert Einstein**

Incoming medical students are selected based on academic performance in college. While the intellectual level of the students is universally high, not surprisingly, humanistic values and social skills, interpersonal attributes difficult to assess from a college transcript and impossible to test on a written exam, vary widely.

Your Doctors' Manners Matter

There is hope for those physicians needing instruction in the language of manners as it applies to their patients. Dr. William T. Branch, Jr., a professor of medicine at Emory University School of Medicine, demonstrated that faculty members who were coached on issues such as how to listen carefully, how to be a caring person, and how to use personal and social information in patient care were better at teaching these skills to medical students than faculty who had not been coached. Interviewed by *The New York Times*, Dr. Branch pointed out that the skills taught to the faculty "can help physicians grow, not just in terms of knowing more but in becoming a whole person."[13]

Reflecting on his own hospital care, Dr. Michael Kahn, a psychiatrist writing in the May 2008 issue of *The New England Journal of Medicine*, noted that while compassion is preferred, most patients would be well served with a doctor who is well behaved. He wrote about his doctor:

> I found the Old World manners of my European-born surgeon—and my reaction to them—revealing in this regard. Whatever he might actually have been feeling, his behavior—dress, manners, body language, eye contact—was impeccable. I wasn't left thinking 'What compassion.' Instead I found myself thinking, 'What a professional,' and even (unexpectedly) 'What a gentleman.' The impression he made was remarkably calming, and it helped to

confirm my suspicion that patients may care less about whether their doctors are reflective and empathetic than whether they are respectful and attentive.[14]

Dr. Kahn goes on to describe a checklist, similar to the ones used by doctors and nurses when performing bedside procedures, to be used when first approaching a patient. As he pointed out, it is easier to modify behavior than to change attitudes. Commenting on the best way to teach behavior to the student doctor, he writes, "Trainees are likely to learn more from watching colleagues act with compassion than from hearing them discuss it." Dr. Kahn includes in his prescription for better care the requirement that physicians be trained to pay attention to the patient. Listening, demonstrating attention to the patient's story, and engaging in a back-and-forth conversation are all dimensions of good manners.

While medical training is long and difficult, very little time is devoted to teaching bedside behavior. The typical primary care physician spends seven to eight years in medical school and residency training before starting in practice, and the training periods for subspecialists can last as long as eleven years. Training is so demanding that medical schools and residency training programs are required by law to set limits on the trainee working hours so they do not become exhausted or overextended.

Your Doctors' Manners Matter

In almost every other field, real life experiences interrupt or end formal training. Adults barely out of their teens learn how to conduct relationships and how to behave in business situations from mentors much older and experienced than they, and from their peers by observing errors. Given the peer group and age of the non-medical school bound college graduate, errors are forgiven and for the successful, not repeated. Medical students, because of their cloistered education, minimal socialization with peer groups outside of medicine, and mentoring by authority figures usually little older than they, remain socially challenged when they are finished with their training.

Medical schools have begun to recognize these deficiencies. Professors do lecture on the essentials of professional bedside behavior, and some medical schools have initiated courses on humanistic values including required readings in fiction and essays. Doctors-in-training are encouraged to present their patients in a humanistic manner rather than as a compilation of symptoms and diseases. They are taught in medical ethics lectures what is right and wrong in terms of medical conduct. What is not taught is how the practitioner should behave in a manner that indicates to the patient what Dr. Calhoun calls the "moral attitudes of respect, tolerance, and considerateness." They are not taught the non-verbal behaviors that demonstrate respect for the dignity of the patient, the nurse, or the colleague.

No other professional has the responsibility to ask for permission to poke and prod, elicit pain, or explore the most intimate areas of the body to help another individual. Out of context, such behavior would be criminal. This unique privilege makes the clear display of manners necessary to place the behavior in context and reassure the patient of the physician's essential moral character. Medical manners communicate, in everyday behavior, the principles of medical ethics.

Good manners signifying respect for the patient can be taught to both students and teachers. Dr. Kahn has it right when he emphasizes polite behavior over feelings. This is because conduct can be taught, behavior can be mimicked, and manners are teachable.

Chapter Three
Behavior of the Effective Physician
Issues Addressed in this Chapter

- Good manners are a core value of good medical care.//
- Good manners foster good communication.
- After a consultation with the doctor you should feel like you have expressed your fears, told your story, and you and the doctor are in agreement as to what is the problem.
- Ordering a lot of tests is not a substitute for listening to a patient's story.
- Trust is established by face-to-face time with your physician.
- Acting in a way that shows respect for you as a patient and a human being is the mark of an excellent doctor.
- If your doctor is not listening, be assertive, share your concerns.

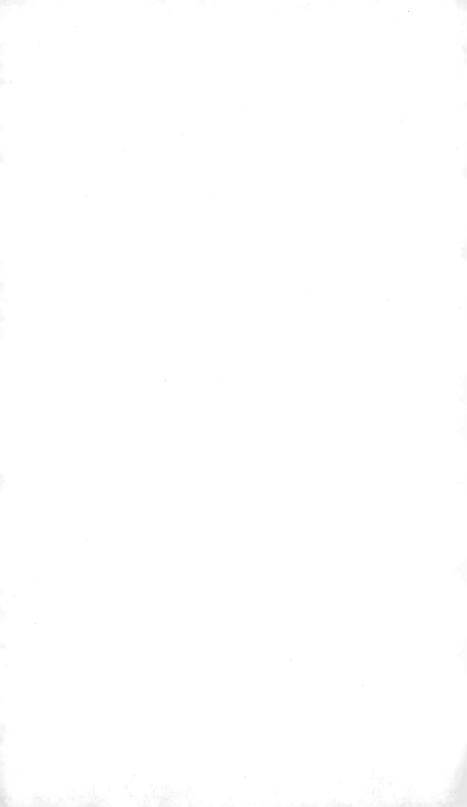

SECTION TWO
Finding the Right Doctor

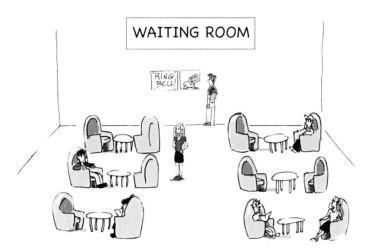

Chapter Four

The Office Consultation

To write prescriptions is easy, but to come to an understanding with people is hard.

– Franz Kafka, "A Country Doctor," 1919

Your first scheduled visit to the doctor's office as an independently living adult is often prompted by an employer, an insurance company, or a concerned spouse or significant other. For many women, if they have not already visited an obstetrician-gynecologist for a physical exam, the first visit is for a Pap smear or a prenatal evaluation, or a visit may follow a referral after an emergency department visit.

If your visit is a response to an injury or illness, in all likelihood you will take with you an opinion of what condition is causing your symptoms. This opinion is strongly influenced by family, friends, and any information you are able to access. Perhaps your mother-in-law has arrived at a diagnosis and wonders if the doctor will agree with her and care for you to her satisfaction. The person you live with probably has some idea of what illness your symptoms point to, and your friends may have insisted they can save you a trip to the doctor if you will just take the same vitamins they do. Then there is all that information and those questionable stories and opinions you have discovered on the Internet. All those opinionated, self-appointed experts, although invisible, are in the examining room with you as you strip to the buff. However, only you bring to the consultation a full knowledge of your problem, your symptoms, and how they affect your life.

You know the most about your body, and you know the reason why you have sought out the consultation. In many cases, that reason is not necessarily the symptom, but has more to do with what you believe the symptom means. After all, chances are pretty good that mole on your stomach is not all that bothersome, but if a family member died of skin cancer, you start to examine the mole carefully in the mirror, searching for changes in shape, color, or size. Is it really bigger, or darker, or is the border less regular? You are not sure, but you sure are worried.

That pain in your shoulder doesn't hurt except when you swing a tennis racket. This will not interfere with your usual activities, but since the league season is about to start, you are concerned you will not be able to play.

The backache you've been experiencing for the past several weeks is not all that severe, but you are on your feet all day at your job, and your coworker just had spinal surgery and was out for three weeks. This is not something you can afford. It's not just the symptom, but also how the symptom will affect your life that brings you to the doctor's office.

What You Want and What You Get

You want your doctor to take time for explanations and to ask about and pay attention to your main concern. You want your doctor to become involved in your care and to show concern for your health by asking what worries you the most and why. You also have some expectations of what the doctor will do or say, and you may be right, somewhat off base, or totally misinformed. As David Pendleton and colleagues point out, any consultation that fails to take into account your expectation is likely to lead to a less than optimal outcome and will be unsatisfactory to you and your doctor.

The doctor demonstrates his concern by treating you with courtesy and engaging you in a conversation about your problem. Isn't it true that when someone sits and listens to you tell your story, appears interested, and wants to learn more, your estimation of their character and wisdom increases? In any other setting, if you wanted to dominate a conversation by discussing your health, you would be cut off as a bore, but when the doctor sits and listens, leans forward, eyes wide, interrupting only for clarification and then only when necessary to keep you on track, you get the feeling of interest and caring. The doctor listens to your ideas, feelings, and concerns, and discovers how you have coped with the problem up to that point. In an effective consultation, the doctor gains an awareness of what your symptoms are and how they affect your daily activities, and you gain an understanding of the nature of your problem and what it will take to relieve your discomfort and return to your usual state of health.

A polite and agreeable doctor is more likely to do a better job at communicating recommendations, and you will do a better job following them. While it's true that the doctor is not seeing patients at their best—pain and discomfort have a way of bringing out the worst in us and doctors being human, a sullen or surly patient can affect even the most professional demeanor—if you perceive your doctor as a courteous professional with a positive outlook about your condition, you are more likely to relax, have a more positive outlook, and you will feel more satisfied with the consultation.

In his book, Dr. Jerome Groopman writes, "We all want to feel that our physician really likes us, sees us as special, and is emotionally moved by our plight, attracted not so much by the fascinating biology of our disease but by who we are as people."[1] The doctor who demonstrates empathy and communicates an intense desire to provide the best possible care will get the best results.

Although medical school curricula have recently recognized the need to include courses in medical literature as a way of exposing students to the ideas of empathy and compassion in the healing arts, the messages trainees receive are mixed. Doctors-in-training are also taught to remain emotionally detached from their patients because emotional involvement can color decision making, cause burnout, and can result in inaction when a life-saving maneuver requires a life-endangering procedure. Emotional involvement can even lead to inappropriate social interactions. However, good manners and courteous behavior do not get in the way of excellent professional judgment and medical care.

Is It Safe?

Even in the best of circumstances, personalities influence the interaction between doctor and patient in a way that can undermine the effectiveness of the visit. For example, you may think of the doctor as an authority figure, and this can influence the way the two of you communicate. By virtue of training, education, and role in society, the medical doctor enjoys a unique position in a community. Only the medical doctor has the honorific used in routine social situations, the medical doctor is sought out in emergencies, and in most cases, the medical doctor is financially stable.

The nature of the consultation makes the doctor's apparent authority even more obvious. At some point, you will be subjected to a close inspection of your body. You might feel as if the doctor is being critical rather than analytical, or that you are being judged. It's almost impossible for this not to occur when one person is naked or nearly so, the other fully dressed. The power dynamic under these conditions is so obvious, it is a technique used by some military intelligence groups. Add to this the orders you are given—sit on the table, turn on your side, sit up, lie down, take a deep breath, don't breathe—orders you willingly follow. If you are in pain—think of Dustin Hoffman's character sitting in the dentist's chair in *Marathon Man*—it is natural to feel at least a little intimidated.

If you think of your doctor as an authority figure instead of a professional helping you solve a problem, you may respond in a number of unhelpful ways. You may succumb and become passive, expecting the doctor to be able to figure out all he needs to know. After all, he is the authority and you are "just" a patient. You might feel less willing to fully discuss the symptoms and the treatment options available to you, and what you have to contribute is not important. Guard against this. Studies have shown passive patients who fail to participate actively in the consultation will suffer a failure in treatment more often than the actively involved patient. Although your office visit may proceed smoothly, you will be less likely to follow the treatment protocol if you don't feel like you had a hand in planning it.

Working Together

As David Pendleton and colleagues write in their book, the most successful physician visit is a collaboration between equals. The physician has expertise about the science of medicine and you, the patient, are an expert on how you are affected by your symptoms and the limitations your environment places on your ability to follow the doctor's treatment recommendations. On follow-up, only you know how well any prescribed treatments are working to improve your feelings of well-being. Let's see how well the collaboration works in the following true story. As in all our patient narratives, the names and institutions have been changed.

* * *

Martha W. considers herself a successful businesswoman, wife, and mother. She has a rewarding career as a real estate agent. She is always near the top of her office in sales. She understands the importance of satisfying customers and is proud of her knowledge of the market. Skillful at identifying her clients' needs, she works hard to also satisfy their desires. She appreciates the importance of being on time and well prepared for appointments. Having sold homes to new physicians just beginning their practices and to established physicians enjoying financial success, she is comfortable around doctors and appreciates their long hours and difficult work schedules.

Bothersome abdominal cramps and bowel irregularity prompted a visit to her internist, a physician she had been seeing for twenty years. Her internist referred her to Dr. Mark Glenn, a gastroenterologist in a large subspecialty group. Dr. Glenn enjoyed a wide reputation among his colleagues as an excellent diagnostician and for his knowledge and skill in the endoscopy laboratory.

On calling his office for the appointment, Martha was advised to be early in order to complete the necessary paperwork. Here is how she tells the story.

"When I made the appointment by phone, I was asked by the doctor's assistant to arrive forty-five minutes early to fill in insurance and history intake forms, which I did. The sign-in sheet was unattended in front of a closed, clouded glass window labeled "Reception." I filled in the requested information and waited another fifteen minutes before I saw any of the doctor's staff. The office furniture looked old and worn, the magazines were laughably ancient, and anyway, the room was so dimly lit and the TV so loud, I could not have read. Finally the receptionist appeared and asked me to fill in an eight-page form asking for my health insurance, current complaints, past medical history, and any other problems I might be having and medication I was taking.

"When they finally called me, I had been in the office for an hour. They placed me in a small exam room, gave me a paper gown, and asked me to completely undress. I waited another thirty minutes in that chilly room for Dr. Glenn. He wore a scrub suit, wrinkled and stained on the front with what I hoped was catsup, and a soiled lab coat that was probably white at one time, but now had a dull gray tint. The sleeves of his lab coat had both mustard and catsup on the edges.

"He seemed rushed. He did not offer his hand, and I don't think he smiled once during my exam. Instead of coming over to the exam table, he went immediately to a computer, sat down in front of it, and alternated flipping through the forms I had filled out and tapping on the keyboard. After a few minutes, he asked me how long I had my symptoms and what medicines my family doctor had put me on. Then he asked me many questions about the pain, how long I had been on the two drugs, had I lost weight, was I having any emotional issues. All in less than five minutes, all without looking up from the computer. I didn't have time to think about my answers, but it was on the form anyway, except the emotional issues.

"Then he asked me to lie down and the gown opened up. I was embarrassed and said the gown doesn't work well. Not that I meant to complain. I just wanted him to know I'm not an exhibitionist. He looked at me like I was an idiot and told me I put it on wrong, that it opens in the back. Now I was not only embarrassed, I felt stupid. Then without a word he started to poke my belly here and there, asking me if it hurt. I tried to tell him his hands hurt, but if he was trying to get the pain to come back, he didn't. He said, 'Unh hunh, unh hunh,' but I'm not sure he understood.

"I will say he was very thorough in his exam, but he did not say anything about the lump he found in my groin despite spending an inordinate amount of time examining it, a lump I didn't even know I had. After finishing the exam, he went back to the desk and restarted tapping into the computer. Finally, he looked up at me and told me to get dressed. I don't think I have been naked for that long since my honeymoon, if then. The gown was ripped in several places, and what I really wanted to do was dress in private. I mean, how do you have a conversation when you are stark naked except for a few paper tatters and standing in front of a man who is completely dressed?

'We're going to have to run a bunch of tests,' he said.

'What are you looking for?' I asked.

'It would take too long to explain it, and anyway, the only important thing is what we find.'

"Apparently my condition was top secret, and I was on a need-to-know classification.

'And what do you think that will be?' I asked.

'I can't really say until we run all the tests. My nurse will schedule the procedures and blood work and answer any questions.'

"Procedure? No one mentioned any procedure. I didn't want to talk to the nurse. I wanted to talk to the doctor. He was the one who had poked his gigantic finger up my butt.

"Then he wrote out two prescriptions but never really told me how to take them or what they were for, and by this time I was too intimidated to ask. I had to ask the pharmacist."

* * *

Martha left the office anxious, angry, confused, discouraged, and frustrated. What should she do? A physician she trusted had referred her; other physicians she knew attested to the consultant's knowledge and skill. Her confidence in the specialist had been high when she entered his office, but his physical appearance, the office environment, the behavior of the staff, and most significantly, the physician's manners alienated her. Not only that, she felt she had failed to convey all the information the specialist needed to make a full diagnosis.

She never returned for the procedures and instead asked her internist to refer her to another doctor. The time and money spent on the visit was wasted, Martha's problem was no better, her faith in her long-time internist was tested—he had to apologize for the referral—and Martha's opinion of doctors and the medical care system in general suffered a blow. After all, this was "the best doctor" in town for her problem.

Dr. Glenn did not seem to have time to listen, and he is not alone. The art of listening to patients is being discarded by medical practitioners as a quaint technique taught to medical students and then ignored in medical practice. Some doctors consider a full patient history and a complete physical exam unnecessary, an ancient practice of the last century. After all, these doctors might argue, an automated blood test on a sample as small as $1/30^{th}$ of an ounce (about 1 cc) and medical images once regarded as the stuff of science fiction can tell the doctor in a few seconds what might take an hour to figure out by listening and examining the patient. In our opinion, relying solely on technology to care for a patient is expensive, dangerous, and impersonal.

The loss of the patient narrative represents more than just discarding an inexpensive but effective diagnostic technique. Martha did not come to the office to receive a slip for blood tests and medication. She wanted to engage the doctor in her problem and have him care about her symptoms. Martha was looking for information given with empathy and compassion or at least with good manners. She left angry and feeling abused.

It is not enough for your doctor to be bright, well trained, and experienced. F. W. Peabody, a legendary physician of the early twentieth century and active in the founding of the renowned Harvard Unit at the Boston City Hospital, wrote in a famous 1927 essay, "One of the essential qualities of the clinician is interest in humanity, the secret of the care of the patient is in caring for the patient."[2]

Martha's treatment in the waiting and reception area, the level of housekeeping, the demeanor of the staff—all seemingly minor niceties—had health consequences. Then she met Dr. Glenn. He communicated his attitude toward his patient through his actions: inattentive listening, unwelcoming demeanor, and treating Martha as "just another patient." True or not, it seemed as if he did not care if Martha followed his recommendations.

Listening to the patient's story is both good manners and good medical practice. When it comes to medical care, attentive listening can make the difference between getting a diagnosis right or wrong, or as in Martha's case, can seriously influence the willingness of the patient to proceed with further tests and stick to a medical regimen.

The extra consideration and planning that could have resulted in learning more about Martha's condition, and in Martha's understanding of the role of the prescribed medication and tests was missing from her visit. As a result, she failed to follow up. Fortunately, she had a good relationship with her internist and went back to him for additional care, but she could just as easily opted out of the medical care system and resorted to self-diagnosis and self-treatment, delaying appropriate therapy.

First Impressions

There are no courses in medical school on managing a medical office. The lessons learned by the hospitality industry, and almost every consumer oriented industry in America—say hello and thank you, be thoughtful and courteous, and care about the consumer's feelings and opinions—have not been carried over to the medical office. In its place is the attitude that only medical knowledge and skills matter.

Your Doctors' Manners Matter

In medical schools, the idea that the patient always comes first is drilled into the student doctors, but what they are taught and what happens in practice are often different. Doctors' offices operate under conflicting pressures. As every retail operation knows, the customer must be happy, but who is the customer? You, the patient, of course, or maybe the insurance company, or even the hospital or outpatient surgery center where patients are referred. The reality is the profession is ambivalent. There is a disconnect between the business bottom line in the delivery of your medical care and your comfort and any inconvenience you may suffer.

One important way the doctor can demonstrate a willingness to listen to your concerns is by providing an office that is welcoming. It has been our sad personal observation that this goal is rarely met. Your first contact with the office is a phone call to make the appointment. Although cost considerations make the use of an automated telephone system a necessity, no one wants to leave a message about an intimate problem on an answering machine. The new patient should be able to quickly bypass the system and speak with an empathetic, unhurried attendant. Your doctor's credibility as an empathetic and caring practitioner will suffer a big hit if your first contact with the office is no more personal and no less frustrating than a computerized help line.

Consider your mood when the waiting room is extremely plain and uninviting, the reception staff is curt and unfriendly, or the wait is long with no effort made to inform you of the reason or the time until you will be seen. The medical office, along with the Department of Motor Vehicles and the jury waiting room, are among the few places left in our modern, consumer-oriented society where the average person will routinely encounter employees acting in an offhanded, indifferent, or rude and disrespectful manner, and where a work-related goal appears to be unpleasant personal encounters. Once you see the physician, you are not likely to be fully communicative, especially so if the nurse is rude or the doctor rushed.

A long delay until the day of the appointment or a further delay while sitting in the waiting room can make even the most cooperative of patients irritable, unresponsive, and less likely to accept a doctor's recommendations. If you do feel yourself becoming irritable because of a delay, either discuss your feelings openly with the appointment clerk or nurse and see what can be done for you, or take a deep breath and a mental time-out.

Not surprisingly, the furnishings of many medical offices reflect the attitude of the folks who work in them. Some waiting rooms are bleak islands of poor taste bordering on dreadful décor—drab, cold, and uninviting.

Your Doctors' Manners Matter

The attitude of the personnel and the often depressing character of the patient surroundings can affect your willingness to communicate your most personal problems and may give you some doubt concerning the attention the doctor will give to your concerns.

Physical comfort in the office is also important. The waiting room can be a warm and friendly place, with comfortable seating, some decorative flourish without excess, and no medical equipment. Patient educational material is appropriate. Chairs can be grouped around reading material on tables and in bookcases rather than arranged in rows and columns facing the office staff. The clerical functions of a doctor's office do not make for interesting theater and should be screened from patient view.

The office should have adequate numbers of well-supported armchairs. Couches appear luxurious, but if you are in pain, they will be uncomfortable. Televisions do distract the nervous, but a TV screen is impossible to ignore. An ideal arrangement is to place the TV about ten feet from and facing a wall, with a grouping of chairs between the wall and the screen. The TV should be mounted, but not so high that the sound needs to be turned up. The dates of issue of the magazines should not be a cause for ridicule. Healthcare magazines and taped programs about healthcare topics are appropriate.

Your name should not be called from a door twenty feet away. This is rude and embarrassing in a crowded waiting room. In a large practice with a common waiting area, a system of grouping patients by doctor or time slot will allow the nurse to come within a few feet of the patient before calling out a name. Even better, taking a lesson from restaurants, you can be notified by a text message on your cell phone or be given a local area pager. A nice courtesy is for the nurse to escort the patient from the waiting area to the next stop on the journey, with the patient setting the pace. Do not be embarrassed to ask for a wheelchair. You are in a doctor's office; they are used to managing wheelchairs, although on occasion the staff may forget to ask if you would like one.

Any previous records of visits to the same office should be complete and immediately available. A well-designed computer system will serve to reach this goal. You can help in this regard. If you have been referred by another doctor, or if you have hospital records, or if you have lab work or X-rays not ordered by the doctor you are about to see, we strongly advise that you take the time to obtain a copy and hand carry these with you to your appointment. Do not trust reassurances that the information has been sent—not from your referring doctor, not from the lab, and definitely not from the hospital. It may or may not have been sent, it may or may not make it to your newly created file in the consulting doctor's records, or it may be with all those other lost records, floating in another dimension, a huge nebulae of medical information caught in a black hole in the universe. An alternative is to check with the doctor's office to see if your records have arrived before your visit. If they are not there, redouble your efforts to have the records sent.

You are entitled to be addressed by your proper honorific and family name: Mrs. Smith, Ms. Jones, Dr. Johnson, Mr. Brown. You may have to express your preference more than once. Do not be shy about this. The staff is there to make you feel comfortable and many patients, especially if there is a huge age difference between them and the staff or the doctor, prefer formal forms of address. It shows respect. We all know life's not easy. Not everyone will survive your number of years, and if nothing else, that should be honored. If you prefer first name use, you can make this known as well.

Waiting, Waiting, Waiting

Many offices run late, and this may be unavoidable. However, as Miss Manners writes in her book *Miss Manners' Guide to Excruciatingly Correct Behavior*, "it is uncivilized, wicked, unconscionable, barbarous, and unethical the way the medical profession [habitually] keeps patients waiting."[3] Judith Martin comments (sarcastically, we hope) "that doctors have so much in the way of the world's riches that it is not necessary for them to have manners." She implies that the practice of medicine is organized in a way that makes rude behavior the norm.

As the French say, "Men count up the faults of those who keep them waiting." Sharon Schwarze, writing in the *Journal of Clinical Ethics* in an article "Being on Time for Appointments," indicates it is not only unethical and disrespectful to be late, being late for an appointment breaks a binding oral agreement.[4]

There are, to be fair, many reasons the physician may run late. These might include unexpected delays in starting or completing procedures, medical emergencies, the late arrival of scheduled patients, unforeseen phone calls from the hospital or patients, and there are more. What is not acceptable is poor office management, over scheduling, and inconsiderate and contemptuous concern for your time.

The office staff can help. They should keep you posted as to how late the doctor is likely to be. A general explanation of the reason reduces frustration. A savvy office worker avoids explanations such as the doctor is busy, or at lunch, or had a hard night. Explanations such as a patient needs extra attention or care, or a patient emergency has arisen, or one of the doctor's colleagues needs your doctor's special expertise for an emergency situation. (Even we are impressed by that one when we are waiting.) You want your doctor to give priority to a patient who requires immediate care to prevent

Your Doctors' Manners Matter

permanent disability or a worsening condition. If a significant delay is expected, and significant is a relative term, the staffer should offer you a new appointment, if practical, rather than have you wait longer than is possible given your schedule.

There are some things you can do to reduce your chances at being stuck, or limit your frustration if you are. Try to make the first appointment in the morning or the afternoon. It is generally a good idea not to schedule anything important or dependent on timing around a doctor's appointment. That means someone else should do carpool. Also, it is generally a good idea to bring along your own reading material; we recommend an engaging novel or collection of short stories.

Other general courtesies are to wear minimal or no perfume or cologne. Keep conversation in a low voice. If you must use your cellphone, leave the waiting area for a corridor if possible. Let someone on the staff know where you are.

Face Time

When the doctor arrives, he or she will continue taking a history, face-to-face, by asking questions about your symptoms and your past medical history. The dialogue that follows can be conducted in two general ways. Some doctors will ask a question such as "what brought you here" and often the response is something like "I've got a cold."[**] This is really a self-diagnosis and many doctors at this point will interrupt and ask a number of questions trying to prove or disprove this diagnosis. This technique of interrupted direct questioning can lead to dissatisfaction for the doctor and the patient. Many patients will feel as if they have not been given a chance to tell their story. An alternative method is for the doctor to allow you to speak, directing you into a focused narrative or story of your illness by asking more open-ended questions, such as what else is bothering you, what does your spouse think is wrong or how have you been dealing with this problem, and what do you think will help and why.

Listening to a complete history is an important tool for the doctor to arrive at a diagnosis. If, for whatever reason, you are not telling your story quite like you want to—it happens—the doctor may ask an open-ended question to help you focus. Such questioning results in higher levels of patient satisfaction, no or limited increases in time spent during the consultation, and a perception on your part of having spent more time with the doctor.

[**] An old joke about taking a history is the following:
The doctor walks into the examining room.
Doctor: "So. What brought you here today, Mr. Smith?"
Mr. Smith: "The midtown bus."

Your Doctors' Manners Matter

If you have been interrupted, say something like: "I'll get to that in a second, but first…" If you forgot what question you were answering initially, or what you were saying, say "now where was I?" or "I'm sorry, what was that first question? I hadn't finished answering." That'll slow down the questions, and chances are the follow-up will change based on your completed story. Telling your story in your own words and in your own time leads to a more thorough evaluation and a better chance at an accurate diagnosis.

However, keep in mind that time is precious to the doctor and there is never enough of it. If the doctor spends an extra five minutes for each patient, and she sees twenty patients a day (not a lot), that's more than an extra hour and a half in the office. Ouch. So be prepared when you come to the doctor. Have a list of questions. If it's clear your concerns will take a lot of time, ask the doctor if you can schedule a second visit just to discuss them.

Open-ended questions asked in the final phase of the consultation, and before you and the doctor discuss the diagnosis and the treatment plan, will clarify your main concerns and allow the doctor to address them directly. An example would be: "Is there anything you are concerned about that we have not discussed?" Two questions your doctor should avoid asking are "do you have any other questions" and "is there anything else I can do for you." These are the questions help-line operators use and the underlying message is: "This conversation is over." Before the consultation ends, try to remember to take a deep breath and repeat back to the doctor what you understand and ask about what you do not.

By the end of the consultation, you should feel you have told the complete story of your illness, and you have communicated your fears. You should also get the feeling that the doctor is interested and empathetic. If the doctor fails to get a complete history, treatment will likely be incorrect. If you leave the office feeling the doctor was not empathetic, you will likely ignore the advice.

Open-ended questioning can be more satisfying for the doctor as well. Not surprisingly, when asking the same questions about different symptoms, and hearing similar responses from different patients, doctors voice the complaint that they see the same old thing every day. Open-ended interviews can reveal needed information as well as interesting stories, making history-taking more satisfactory for the doctor.

In some offices, you may be asked to undress in the exam room before the doctor comes in to take a history. This is done to save time. Unfortunately your ability to provide a full response may be inhibited by the fact that you are practically naked.

The physical exam will follow. Any unexpected findings on exam will stimulate additional questions. Upon completion of the exam, the doctor can usually arrive at a diagnosis, or if not, then a plan to obtain more information through tests or consultations with specialists.

The exam room, where you will disrobe, should be kept warmer than the offices and waiting area. It goes without saying that the offices should be spotless and the examining room tidied after each patient. However, lighting is sometimes ignored. The offices in general should be well lighted and cheerful, but the exam room should be bright. Although privacy in the waiting area is a challenge, there is no excuse for a lack of privacy once you have entered the back offices and exam area.

In many practices, the consultation is completed in a separate office, after the physical exam, where the patient and doctor discuss results and plans. Often the doctor will decorate this office with framed diplomas and honors received. The office is the place for reference books and a computer so that the doctor can access an article or quickly research a particular question. These sources can also serve the purpose of patient instruction. Take a good look at your doctor's desk. An overly large desk is a barrier rather than a piece of furniture bringing two experts together.

An efficient office staff will prevent you from feeling rushed or interrupted. This means scheduling should be realistic, calls should be managed, a personal cellphone ignored and the doctor's manner unhurried and bright. Interruptions affect the thinking process and communication. You may forget to mention a problem, or feel you are intruded upon. As a patient, you do not have control over this potential problem, other than to try to schedule your visit as the first in the morning or after the staff breaks for lunch.†† Keep in mind that both you and the doctor value your time together, so try to stay focused in your questions and attentive to the responses. However, do not hesitate to ask about issues you find confusing or to voice concerns you believe are unique to your situation.

Keep your cellphone in the off position. This is time you have reserved. You cannot expect the doctor's complete attention if you do not give your complete attention to the consultation.

Up to the point where you and the doctor are sitting across his desk from each other, you have been the expert, providing information to him about your illness. Now the information flows in two directions. The doctor gives you an opinion as to why you are ill, the choices you have for dealing with your illness, and the rationale for a treatment plan. You provide information as to what you can realistically do, and what you will need help

---

†† Many doctors do not take a true "lunch break." There are patients to see in hospital, calls to make to colleagues, and insurance company busywork that must be done.

with. Finally, you and the doctor reach a decision as to how to proceed. It is in the final part of the consultation that you should ask all your questions and expect answers.

Dr. Barbara Korsch, a professor of Pediatrics at USC, has studied the consultation process throughout her career. She terms the education part of the consultation a "joint venture." She points out that during this part of the consultation, your needs for information as well as what you think is needed must be addressed and the information given to you must be relevant.[5]

Speak freely. If you do not communicate to the doctor what you believe is making you ill, then the doctor must feel out what you need explained. Your ideas about your illness may not be correct, but if you fail to discuss them, or the doctor fails to take those ideas into consideration, it is likely you will leave the office dissatisfied and unlikely to follow the recommendations.

As we saw with Martha W., satisfaction with the consultation is critical to following the treatment plan. Patient adherence is one of the main goals of the medical consultation. In the medical journal *British Journal of General Practice*, the researcher Dr. Glyn Elwyn summarizes the doctor's tasks necessary to achieve patient compliance or adherence.[6] If the consultation is considered a team effort, with you and the doctor working to reach a successful conclusion to the consultation, your tasks might look like the following:‡‡ Tell the doctor why you called for the appointment. Do not be embarrassed. You are there to be helped, not judged. Discuss how the problem affects you and what you think might help. Consider carefully the doctor's opinion and restate it in your own words to prove you understand what you heard. Come to an agreement as to what the problem is. With complex problems, this can become a negotiation. Be open. Respond thoughtfully. Make sure you have listened carefully; make sure the doctor understands your special needs and that you can carry out the instructions once you leave the office. Before you leave, be sure you understand by repeating in your own words the information you are given, especially about medications and follow-up. It is often helpful to have two sets of ears, you and your partner or sibling or good friend, so if you are confused you can review what was said with the person who accompanied you. You should be able to explain what you are expected to do and why. Repeating the information you are given reinforces your commitment to your program and makes it more likely you will follow it. Remember, you will be responsible for the treatment plan. Finally, be sure you are given a sheet of paper with written instructions.[7]

---

‡‡ Much of the following is adopted from Pendleton, et al and Elwyn, et al.

Your Doctors' Manners Matter

You may be under great strain and dealing with difficult conditions at home or at work that complicate your ability to follow the recommended treatment. Discuss these with your doctor and any appropriate staff. They are there to help you. Be polite, even in the face of less than civil behavior on the part of the staff. Especially in the face of less than civil behavior.

The majority of professionals we have worked with in the medical or allied profession have a desire to help people feel better. A confident and buoyant doctor and staff can go a long way to encouraging you to adopt treatment recommendations. However, anyone can have a bad day. It is not always easy to be cheerful when dealing with death and disease. Any rudeness you encounter is not likely to be deliberate, and confronting bad manners with polite behavior sets an example.

Work to establish a pleasant relationship, even though the circumstances may be difficult. It will help you achieve your goal. Never confront a rude office worker. You might make matters worse. If you have an unpleasant experience, after you leave the office a polite personal note to the doctor about an embarrassing or stressful encounter will serve to raise the awareness of the individuals involved. Do this even if the doctor was the involved individual. Be constructive. Do not attack the individual. Concentrate on the situation. You should get a letter or phone call in response. Remember to maintain a positive attitude. This is a teachable moment.

Again. Be polite. Do not write the letter while you are fuming about your mistreatment. Keep in mind that just as you have the freedom to choose a new doctor, the doctor has the freedom to ask you to seek care elsewhere.

Your Doctors' Manners Matter

Chapter Four
The Office Consultation
Issues Addressed in this Chapter

- Be sure to tell your complete story, even if you are interrupted.

- Go into the doctor's office with your questions written down. Take notes when the doctor gives you your instructions.

- Have a friend or family member accompany you to the office.

- Before you leave the consultation, be sure you understand and are in agreement with the doctor's opinion.

- A welcoming office fosters good communication. Let the office staff know how you wish to be addressed.

- If the doctor is delayed, you should be informed of how long you will have to wait and arrangements can be made for another appointment if practical.

- Your doctor should be open to questions about cost and other social issues as it affects your care.

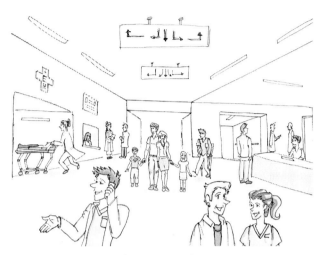

Chapter Five

The Hospital Experience

Mrs. Cushing: *I think one of your patients in here is dead, Dr. Spezio.*
Dr. Spezio: *Why do you say that, Mrs. Cushing?*
Mrs. Cushing: *Because he wouldn't give me his Blue Cross number, Dr. Spezio.*

– From the movie *The Hospital*, 1971

Your stay in the hospital will be a unique experience with the potential to be transformative or nightmarish. Despite the unfamiliar environment and potentially disorienting schedule, of one thing you are certain. You are in the hospital to receive the best possible care. This is your goal. To achieve that goal every person involved in your care—the doctors, nurses, and other healthcare personnel—must operate as a team. Time, schedules, assigned duties, and skills all must be coordinated into a unified effort. You are a member of this team—the newest member. You have an assigned role, that of the patient, and if your stay in the hospital is to be successful, the hospital staff must help you be a part of the team.

The problem is, you have no idea what your duties are and how best to carry them out. Well, relax. That is your first duty. Many patients suffering from chronic conditions or pain often comment on a feeling of relief once they are settled into their hospital room. The sheets are clean and taut, the bed is well made, the room may be Spartan, but it is functional, neat, and clean. In all likelihood, a huge carafe of ice water sits on the night table and a pleasant and efficient nurse is on hand to greet and orient you to your surroundings. The staff is there to help you in every way—from the most basic biologic function to the most complex family interactions. If you have a medical, social, or personal problem, there is someone on the staff who knows how to deal with it and wants to help.

Care is centered on you, the patient, and the staff will try their best to coordinate your care, minimize interruptions to your rest, and accommodate your needs. However keep in mind that the hospital staff must meet the needs of all their patients, some more ill than others, some in more distress than others, some less able to care for themselves than others. So your second duty is to cooperate. Try to fit into the hospital routine, and keep in mind that in a hospital, emergencies are a constant, not a rare occurrence. If you are scheduled for a test, it may be delayed or even cancelled for the day because another patient needs the test on an emergency basis.

One patient of ours, the tiniest of premature babies, less than two pounds, developed a life-threatening bowel perforation requiring emergency surgery. All the operating rooms were in use at the time, and it was already late in the day. The one room expected to be freed up was scheduled for a knee replacement. The patient was a fifty-year-old man who had been admitted that morning for the operation and had been waiting his turn.

We had no option. The baby could not wait the two or three hours it would take until another room became free. The man had to be bumped so our baby could get his bowel repaired. This resulted in another three-hour wait for the adult patient, who did not have his surgery completed until ten p.m. that night.

I visited him the next morning. I explained the situation and thanked him for his patience. He remarked that had he been asked, of course he would have volunteered to be bumped.

Delays in the hospital, which sometimes seem interminable, are not a result of capricious decisions, or doctors with late tee times (doctors incur severe penalties if they arrive late to the OR), or a VIP getting preferred treatment. Neither of us has ever seen that happen, and we can assure you the doctor responsible for the care of the bumped patient would register a complaint. A delay is almost invariably the result of an unavoidable rescheduling of the use of the hospital facilities and staff to accommodate those who are most in need. Hospital scheduling is a complex business when events proceed as planned, but once the day gets rolling, scheduling is all about working around emergencies. Your forbearance and understanding will be greatly appreciated by the rest of your team, and when the situation arises, they will watch out for you and go to bat for you.

What to Expect in the Emergency Department

Most visits to the doctor's office are scheduled. However, a hospital admission may be scheduled, such as for a surgical procedure, or due to an emergency, such as a heart attack. Your admission may be through the admissions office and then directly to a room or through the emergency department (ED).

When you enter the ED, a professional member of the medical team who is trained to recognize a critical medical problem must evaluate your complaints. This could be a physician, nurse, or physician's assistant (PA). If your problem is judged to be urgent, it must be addressed immediately before any requests for health insurance are made. This is not a suggestion for good behavior but is mandated by federal law. If the hospital does not meet this requirement, they are subject to a large financial penalty.

The most frequent complaint in the emergency department is the long wait times. If you have a complaint that does not require immediate attention, you should be informed of how long a wait to expect before you will be taken to an exam room.

We often have to wait for service in our daily routines. This is not unique to hospitals. Some public transit systems display the wait time between trains, and you have to take a number in a busy bakery or deli and your position in line is prominently displayed. Hospitals can do this. All it takes is a little communication between the nurses, the reception clerk, and you, the patient. Some hospitals actually post the emergency department wait times on electronic billboards next to highways as an enticement to visit. It cannot be that difficult to communicate the same information when you arrive at the front door.

When you are taken to the exam room, the nurse should inform you when to expect the physician. After you have been evaluated, the physician should tell you what the concerns are, what tests will be necessary to evaluate your problem, and how long it will take to complete those studies. If your physician is called away to an emergency, the staff should keep you informed and let you know when to expect the physician's return.

In most ED examining rooms, your family member can stay with you unless you are in critical condition and receiving immediate life-sustaining therapy. Unruly children create a disturbance, and the small ED examining rooms generally do not accommodate large groups of family and friends.

When you leave the ED, you should receive a written summary of the diagnosis and the results of any completed tests, the doctor's recommendations, written advice and education about any recommended therapies, prescriptions that come with detailed instruction on how to take them and any expected side effects. You should also be given directions to an open pharmacy capable of filling the prescription, or if that is not practical you should be given a sufficient supply until a pharmacy is open and is expected to have the prescription in stock. If you experience a recurrence of your problem, you should receive instructions about what to do and where to go.

You should also receive a recommendation about following up with a physician in an office, or be given the name of a physician who will see you if you do not have

Your Doctors' Manners Matter

one. If you are uncertain about who will provide your follow-up care, you should receive instructions on how to obtain a copy of your medical note. Since many EDs use computerized medical records, you can request a copy of the note to take with you when you leave. You have a right to have copies of your medical records. You may be asked for a nominal charge to cover the copying cost.

We also believe you should receive a summary of the ED fees. The hospital's computer system has that data and at each point of service, personnel are inputting charges before or as they provide the service. Emergency department bills can be quite large, anywhere from hundreds to many thousands of dollars, and many insurance plans place significant responsibility on you to pay. The best time to review and question the charges is when the experience is fresh in your mind. Errors in hospital bills are very common. For example, you may be charged for oxygen or an IV because the physician routinely uses those therapies in patients with your symptoms, except maybe in your situation the severity of your symptoms did not warrant their use, and they were not ordered.

* * *

The following case is an example of an emergency department experience that would have been improved with more attention to the needs of the patient.

When Mark Z. fell off his bike, injuring his arm and shoulder, he went to the nearest hospital ED for care. It was a busy time, and the ED seemed chaotic. After filling out forms detailing his insurance information, a triage nurse evaluated him. His injury was not life threatening, so he had to wait an hour before she escorted him to an examining room, recorded his vital signs, and said a doctor would be in to see him soon. Half an hour later, the doctor came in to the room, interviewed him, and examined his now painfully throbbing arm. The doctor was concerned and ordered blood tests and X-rays, which took another hour to complete. For much of that time, Mark lay in the hall outside of X-ray alone and unattended. Finally, he was returned to the ED where, after another thirty minutes, the doctor returned to say his X-rays did not look good. An orthopedic doctor would have to evaluate his injury. The orthopedist did not arrive for another two hours.

Mark spent eight hours in the ED, much of it alone, in pain, frightened, and hungry. He received multiple tests, and his bill was in the thousands. Most of us would look at this experience and say, "Yes, that's about right. That's the average time and sort of experience you might have when visiting the ED." Because this is the standard, it does not mean you should accept it. In reality, much more could be done to provide comfort and expedite care. In Mark's case, the busy ED schedule was the priority, not his needs. He should have been seen by the triage nurse before filling out any forms. X-rays should have been taken immediately, and the orthopedist should have been called as soon as they were evaluated. While he was waiting, his physical needs should have been inquired after by a nurse or technician.

Never go to the ED alone. You should always have a friend or family member with you. They often can help encourage the ED to expedite your care. If you have a physician, call her and ask her to call the ED and check on you. We are impressed that when the ED staff is aware the personal physician is involved, they are a little more attentive to resolving the situation. If you suspect you may need a specialist like orthopedics for bones, infectious disease for pneumonia and high fevers, or a cardiologist for chest pain, you should ask when you are first evaluated for the specialist to be alerted. When they are aware they may have to go to the ED, they arrive earlier and prepared. It is all about placing you first—not the schedule of the ED, X-ray, or laboratory.

What to Expect in the Hospital

If you are scheduled for an elective surgical procedure—one that does not immediately threaten life or limb and is therefore not an emergency—you might be admitted to the hospital through a designated waiting area. You will then be directed to the pre-operative suite where you will receive help in preparing for your surgery. Following the procedure, you will be taken to a special care area for post-operative recovery. If the surgery or anesthesia is extensive, or your hospital stay is expected to be longer than a full day due to concerns about vital bodily functions or bleeding, you may be moved from the recovery area and admitted to a hospital room for further care.

In the past, most hospital stays were longer than one day and patients undergoing elective surgical procedures were usually admitted the night before for testing and any needed consultations with other specialty physicians, including anesthesiologists. Now testing and consultations are done days before admission, and patients are discharged within twenty-three hours following the procedure unless there are mitigating circumstances, such as the advanced age of the patient or other medical conditions.

In most cases, your hospital stay will be short and the only physicians you will see are your surgeon and the anesthesiologist, if you have surgery, or the physician who admits you if you do not. If your admission to the hospital is for longer than one day, in all likelihood you will be examined by more than one doctor and possibly also visited by non-physician healthcare professionals such as a PA, nutritionist, physical therapist, or occupational therapist. These are specialists who, in the opinion of your personal physician, can provide needed opinions that will shorten your stay, or make your recovery less stressful. They may be asked to assist in your care, either for the reason you were admitted or for other medical or surgical conditions that you had before entering the hospital or that developed subsequently.

Technological advances and controlled trials have resulted in huge improvements in the care patients receive in the hospital and have shortened the time required to treat most conditions. Economic pressures from third-party payers have also resulted in dramatic changes to the way care is delivered, and have had a huge impact on the number of days patients stay in the hospital (length of stay). Twenty years ago, a cardiac bypass surgery patient could expect to spend at least ten days in the hospital. Now that length of stay is down to five. A patient with an uncomplicated appendectomy, a minimum three-day stay twenty years ago, can expect to leave the hospital within twenty-four hours.

Any days in the hospital longer than the length of stay your insurance company is willing to reimburse for a given condition or procedure has to be justified by your physician. In most cases, this is initiated by a phone call from a clerical worker with limited medical training. This is just one of many phone conversations your physician must have with third parties concerning your care. Other limits insurance companies place on your physician include who may consult on your care, how many consults you may receive, what drugs you may be put on when you leave the hospital, approval to order specific tests and procedures and on and on. Interestingly, if Medicare or Medicaid is the third-party payer, far fewer restrictions are placed on the decisions your doctor will make about your care.

Managing a patient in the hospital requires a lot of teamwork and schedule coordination. Doctors do everything possible to optimize the time they spend in the hospital with their patients in order to have time to deal with the unexpected or a new emergency. Your help will be hugely appreciated. Ask your nurse, the doctor's PA, or call the office staff to get a time when the doctor is most likely to make rounds. Try to have a close friend or family member in the room to listen to what the doctor has to say. Four ears are better than two. Note-taking is allowed. Turn off the TV or other entertainment devices when the doctor enters. You do not want to be distracted.

The use of hospital-based physicians, called hospitalists, has affected the way hospitalized patients receive care, a change as revolutionary as many technological and economic changes. Hospitalists are physicians, usually internal medicine specialists certified by the American Board of Internal Medicine, who limit their practice to hospitalized patients. Many if not most primary care physicians, often referred to as PCPs, such as family physicians, office-based internists, and general practitioners, once their patients are admitted, will hand off care to the hospitalists and resume care after discharge. Your personal doctor may visit you while you are in the hospital and may informally consult with the hospitalist, but in the usual situation, when the hospitalist assumes care, he or she is the physician primarily responsible for your medical care. Under the best of circumstances, you will see the same hospitalist every day you are in the hospital. But that is not the usual practice; they work shifts and are frequently rotating on and off the ward.

Nurse practitioners (NPs) or PAs are also used extensively in the hospital. This includes the hospitalist service and the specialists. If you are seeing three or four physicians, you may also be visited by three or four NPs or PAs. Sometimes you will wonder who is in charge, or who is making the decisions about your care. If you feel your care is not proceeding well, raise the issue with your doctor. If this does not improve the situation, you may request another physician in the group or in another group with appropriate subspecialty expertise, to either consult or take over your care. For example, if your hospitalist is managing your infection and your course is not improving, you may request a consultation from an infectious disease expert, or if you have had elective surgery and develop early symptoms of respiratory distress (breathing trouble or a new need for extra oxygen) that is not being acted upon with speed, immediately ask for a visit from the pulmonologist or the ICU doctor.

Before you ask another doctor to consult, be sure you have given your in-hospital doctor a chance to change the way your care is being given. If you wish to change doctors, be sure to have the name of an individual or group you know has privileges at your hospital, and who is willing to assume your care. If you do not have that information, know the type of specialist you would like to see. Hopefully, you have established a good relationship with your nurse (this is very important and more on this later) and he or she can recommend, off the record, a group or a doctor. If you get pushback on your request, do not hesitate to ask to speak to the doctor who is the Physician-in-Chief. This is your life. You only have one.

* * *

The following story is about a woman who thought she had one doctor only to find someone else caring for her. This patient was also near the end of life, a problem that often complicates the hospitalization.

Esther is a ninety-three-year-old woman with severe lung disease on constant oxygen therapy. She had been living in assisted living, but remained mentally alert and involved with family and friends. Suddenly, her oxygen level began to fall, she was more short of breath, losing weight, and just failing to thrive. Her family was very concerned the end was near. Her pulmonologist, Dr. Paul P., whom she dearly loved and had great confidence in, admitted her to the hospital for treatment of suspected pneumonia. Esther had a living will and did not want to be resuscitated if her heart stopped.

After admission to the hospital, Dr. P. never showed up. He had forgotten to inform her he was leaving for a two-week vacation in Italy. He did not tell her who would be responsible for her care or tell the family what his plan of care was. When his partners visited Esther, they did not seem to know her history or have a clear idea about her treatment. The family was never informed when the doctors would round, so someone had to stay at her bedside 24/7—if they were on bathroom break, they could miss the doctor.

Esther wore a red "Do Not Resuscitate" bracelet, which the family and Esther became convinced meant "Do Not Treat." This was because the nurses were often slow to respond to her calls and seemed unconcerned about her critical condition, in addition to doctors who seemed indifferent about her care.

The family called in the family doctor and told him they wanted new specialists and raised their concerns about the nurses. He asked for time to consult with the doctors and the nurses before changing her caregivers. The result was a much more attentive and responsive medical staff. Yes, they had mentally signed Esther off as beyond help. But when their error and lack of concern were brought to their attention, they were quick to understand that death does not occur until we take our last breath. For Esther, that time had not come, and she was working hard to recover. She just needed the help and support of her doctors and nurses.

In all cases, the doctor who has responsibility for your care should visit and speak with you at least once a day. Some groups now use NPs or PAs to make the in-hospital visit and this may work out to your advantage if the PA is knowledgeable and has more time to spend with you than the physician. They should tell you when they plan to round so you can be ready with questions and have family or friends in attendance if you feel the need.

If your doctor asks for a consultation from another colleague, you should have the opportunity to speak with the new doctor as well. You should also know when that doctor starts consulting on your care, and when those consultations end. It may be for one visit, or the consulting doctor may visit daily. If so, you should have the opportunity to speak with the consultant daily. Do not expect your doctor to speak with all the members of your family other than your partner or primary home caregiver. Certain federal regulations, called HIPAA regulations, restrict the information the hospital or doctor is able to provide to anyone not involved in your medical care. You or your partner should transmit any information you want to give to your family.

If your family member or partner requires a meeting with the doctor, it is a very good idea to get the expected time of the doctor's next visit, inform the doctor that your partner will be present for an extended conversation, and have your family member or partner waiting. Alternatively, if your in-hospital doctor has an office-based practice, your family member or partner can schedule an appointment with the doctor at his office. You may need your hospital nurse or social worker to help arrange such a consultation.

If, when your in-hospital doctor or NP visits, you are not able to get the information you need, or if you have not been visited at all, for whatever reason, it is not unreasonable to call the physician with whom you have a personal relationship even though he or she is not responsible for your in-hospital care. It is sad but true, while a doctor may ignore or procrastinate responding to requests for a conversation with a patient, it is less common for the doctor to ignore a request for information from the physician who is *sending* him patients.

Hospital Politics

In most hospitals, the physician staff and the nursing staff are separate organizational entities. That is, doctors do not have the responsibility to fill out job evaluations on nurses and ditto for the nurses toward the doctors. So if you are unhappy with your nurse, you need to inform the nurse supervisor. If you are unhappy with your doctor, you need to inform the doctor and give him or her a chance to make things right. If this does not help, ask to speak with the departmental chairperson or the chief of the medical staff. In some hospitals, usually university hospitals or other teaching hospitals, the doctor is an employee of the hospital. In community hospitals, the doctor is independent and has privileges to work in the hospital but must follow the rules and regulations of the hospital or risk losing those privileges.

If your private physician cares for you in a teaching hospital, you may also receive care from house staff physicians. They are also known as residents and are employed by the hospital or the university affiliated with the hospital. Residents are recent medical school graduates, some with up to five or more years' experience, who are training in a specific specialty. Residents act under the supervision of a teaching physician, usually a senior physician who is a professor in the medical school and has patient care experience. Often the professor is also involved in medical research and may have working with him a physician training in a subspecialty. For example, a general surgeon may be receiving additional training in transplant surgery, or an internist may be studying with an expert in endocrinology. These doctors, often called fellows, have completed their residency and some are certified in their specialty but have elected to take additional training in a focused field of study. Usually the fellow is involved in the senior physician's research project as well as in caring for patients on the senior physician's teaching service. Both the professor and the fellow are usually up-to-date on the latest advances in their field and may know of options for your care not available to the generalist.

We will also mention the medical student. Almost always, in a teaching hospital, you will meet the student or a group of students accompanied by the resident and the senior physician—kind of like pilot fish around a shark or cabinet secretaries around the president. (It depends on the senior physician's demeanor.) There are certainly times and situations where the student's presence may be intrusive, and you may refuse to be seen or examined by the student. This is perfectly acceptable. However, interactions with students give you a chance to influence and mold a young career, and some students are quite savvy and know how to work the hospital system to your benefit. In a teaching hospital, you cannot refuse the care of the residents. They are employed by the hospital. If you do not like the resident, you can ask to be on another resident's service. This is also perfectly acceptable.

Of all the doctors you will meet, the most impressionable and those most likely to treat you with the appropriate respect are the students and residents who have managed to retain their idealism and sense of mission despite the long hours and occasionally demeaning treatment they receive at the hands of some insensitive nurses and senior physicians. If you have a chance, reinforce the polite behavior and civility of a young physician-in-training. The first step toward a profession with good manners may be the kind words you exchange with an impressionable doctor-to-be in your hospital room.

Most hospitals have an office you can contact that will act as your representative if you have a complaint about the care you are receiving. This office may be called the patient representative or ombudsman. If you are having difficulty resolving a problem related to your hospitalization, the personnel in that office are there to act as your representative. They can bring your concern to the appropriate department or person and can negotiate for you. They are willing to deal with any hospital problem, from the food service to billing, from insurance companies to the time and arrangements for discharge. The ombudsman can also assist if you are having a problem with the nursing or medical care you are receiving, but in our experience most problems related to nursing or medical care are best resolved by objectively stating your concerns to the nurse or physician directly, and if that does not work, to the nursing supervisor or physician department chairman respectively.

Your Doctors' Manners Matter

Navigating the Hospital Wards

Nowhere is the exercise of civility and good manners among healthcare workers more important to your health than in the hospital. While it is true that doctors and nurses work together as a team, the hospital, like a military unit, is hierarchical. However, unlike a military unit, two parallel hierarchies function side by side. The origin of orders for the care you are to receive almost always starts with your doctor, and your nurse executes those orders. This means all orders from the doctors and all requests for orders by the nurses are not commands, rather they are requests, albeit some of considerable urgency. A resident doctor with one year's experience may be writing orders to a nurse with twenty years' experience. Conflicts of authority and responsibility do arise. These conflicts must be handled with civility and courtesy. Nurses have the right and responsibility to challenge orders they feel are not in keeping with good medical care, and doctors have the right and responsibility to file complaints about nurses who do not appear to have the necessary skills to do their job. Rarely is either measure necessary.

Multiple doctors participating in your care can also complicate matters. Tuesday's doctor may change the orders from Monday, and one subspecialist may change the orders of a different subspecialist. This is called a turf battle, and when they occur, you are the battlefield. It is important to remember that the vast majority of healthcare workers are dedicated to their profession and the patients under their care. Although as in any discipline conflicts may arise out of pique or personality clashes, in most cases disagreements surface because the members of your health team have differing opinions as to the best possible care for you. Conflicts resulting from turf battles, personality clashes, or mean-spirited individuals are an indication of a dysfunctional organization. Clues that such battles are raging are frequent changes to your healthcare plan (sometimes daily) and denigrating comments, often subtle, by hospital staff about each other either to you or in your presence. These should be reported immediately to senior members of administration or the patient representative.

* * *

Medical care is complex, and it is common to have multiple doctors care for you in the hospital. The problems that arise from this situation are illustrated in this patient experience.

Jimmy B. is a fifty-eight-year-old man admitted to the hospital with fever, cough, and shortness of breath. He also suffers from hypertension and diabetes. In his youth, from fifteen to forty-five years of age, he smoked two packs of cigarettes a day. He still enjoys two to four beers a day and at least a six-pack every day on the weekend (especially during football season). Although his internist treated him for his pneumonia, complications during his hospital course included high blood sugar, a small heart attack, and difficulty urinating. Within the first week in the hospital he was being cared for by the hospitalist, an endocrinologist, a cardiologist, an infectious disease specialist, and a urologist. Each of these physicians worked with a PA, so ten different healthcare providers visited him daily, sometimes at the same time. Not surprisingly, he did not know who ordered what tests or which medications. When he asked the doctor visiting him the results of a test or the reason for a medication, the answer was often, "That is not related to the problem I am treating." He spent a lot of time away from his room undergoing tests. Many of the tests required him to be in a fasting state, so he sometimes went several days without eating a regular meal. The doctors, PAs, nurses, and respiratory therapists interrupted his sleep so often he felt sleep deprived. He was not sure if his pneumonia or his hospital care was making him feel ill.

Jimmy felt like a collection of organs and diseases. When he questioned his cardiologist about his discharge, the cardiologist said one of the other doctors was responsible for that decision. The hospitalist told him the cardiologist and infection disease doctors needed to clear him for discharge before he could go home. There seemed to be no one in charge.

The doctors were not communicating with each other or with the nurses. There were five care plans but no one plan. Finally, his wife demanded a conference with the doctors. She demanded to know who was in charge and who would be responsible for keeping her and her husband up-to-date on his daily progress.

This may be one of the most common and serious problems you will face in the hospital. As we stated at the beginning of the book, getting well is a team effort, but if the team is dysfunctional, your care will suffer. You, your family, or your partner needs to be sure everyone is communicating. It may be your most important responsibility as a team member. Your survival depends on it!

* * *

Just as you will meet a variety of doctors with differing degrees of authority and experience, so you will meet members of the hospital nursing and allied health staff with differing roles. The first nurse you meet when you arrive in your room will probably be the nurse assigned to care for you. This is your primary care nurse and the nurse who will help you through the hospital experience. She will give you pamphlets explaining some of the hospital rules and procedures. She will also show you how to contact her if you need assistance.

Her superior is the floor supervisor or a nurse with a similar title. The floor supervisor may have hands-on participation in your care and will be available to help if you have a special request or need. If you are having a problem with an individual on the nursing service, do not attempt to fix the problem by dealing with the individual. It will not help and will only escalate the conflict. Rather, if something goes wrong and you need to ask for a supervisor, it is the floor supervisor who will be first in line to help you. The floor supervisor reports to a department head, also a nurse, or the director of nursing. If the response from the different levels of nursing supervisors is unhelpful, have a friend or family member go to the administrators' suite, identify themselves, and ask for help.

You may meet a nurse clinician, who may interview you but will not care for you directly, a nursing assistant, also assigned specifically to you, and allied health personnel such as occupational therapists, speech therapists, orthotics specialists (prosthesis), physical therapists, audiologists, and others, most of whom have advanced degrees. Some of the nurses will also have advanced degrees, although the nurse assigned to your care will not. Your nurse will either have graduated from a nursing school or college with a two-year degree and has passed a state licensing test and is a registered RN, or has a four-year college degree in nursing, a BSN. Both will be registered nurses. The nursing supervisor almost always has a BSN, and some of the nurse clinicians will hold a master's degree. Some nurses also have a doctorate degree in nursing. However, most of these nurses are not involved in direct patient care.

With rare exception, all the nurses you meet will be solicitous of your welfare, will act as your advocate in your interactions with other healthcare personnel, and will be polite. If you find your nurse is too familiar, or too formal, let him or her know how you prefer to be addressed.

Like every other organization, hospitals have reduced their staff in an attempt to reduce costs. You will discover the effect this has on your care when you use the buzzer or other communication device to request a visit from your nurse. Expect a delay. Do your best to make every interaction as pleasant as possible. Your nurse should do the same. A polite person is an agreeable person and a person we want to be around.

Being agreeable under difficult circumstances is not easy, and we strongly suggest having someone stay with you in your room as much as possible. When it is possible, have a family member or a friend at your side. Ask them to interact with the nurse if you are not up to it. Ask if your companion may accompany you to tests. This is important, for without an aide or companion, after the test or procedure is over, you might have to wait for a transport back to your room for an unacceptably long period. This is where your friend can help by notifying the doctor or supervisor of your distress, firmly requesting a transfer, or asking for a good reason why you cannot leave the testing area.

When you are finally settled in your room and are aware of your surroundings, you will probably be given a pamphlet that spells out your rights and responsibilities as a patient. Chances are you can also access that document on the hospital's website before you are admitted, if your admission is scheduled, or you can request a copy in the mail. Most hospitals take the document seriously. The nurses will also review with you and your family the rules and regulations that will ease your stay and assist your care. This is important information. Sometimes the nurse is busy, the ward is understaffed, or the orientation is just neglected. Be sure you receive this important information and if necessary, ask your nurse to review it with you and your family.

You have a right to privacy. Everyone should knock before entering your room. When you request assistance, there should be a rapid acknowledgement of the request and an indication of how long it will take to fulfill it. You have a right to some quiet restful time on the ward when you are not undergoing tests. If you are constantly interrupted by housekeeping, dietary, maintenance, respiratory therapy, and multiple other services, you can ask the nurse to schedule times when you will not be interrupted so you can rest and recover. Your illness can be exacerbated by exhausting disturbances and sleep deprivation.

Ask for a tentative schedule of tests or procedures that will require you to be out of the room. Except in emergencies, you should get at least a twelve-hour heads up. You and your family should be aware of everything that is planned for you each day, when it will occur, when you should expect to be out of your room, and when to expect your return. Use the information to schedule a friend or family member to accompany you to the test or procedure, but remember, schedules change with the circumstances.

You should be told when you will receive your medications and what they are each time you receive them. Familiarize your companion with all your medications so he or she can check that what you receive is in fact for you. Having a companion in the room will mean help in getting out of bed to use the commode, rearranging your food tray position as the need arises, raising and lowering the bed, and adjusting the pillows. If you are up to reading, have several books or an electronic device with you.

Some folks pay for so-called private duty nursing. This is usually unnecessary. The nurses who function as private duty nurses or "sitters" are usually not allowed to perform nursing duties such as dispensing medication, hanging IVs, charting vital signs, etc. If possible, a friend or family member is a much better companion.

Upon discharge, the nurse must review with you all of your medications and recommended therapies, like physical therapy or diet instruction, and give you written instructions. Review that material carefully. If you are unclear about these orders, especially if your home medications are different from what you have been taking in the hospital, have the nurse call your physician to clarify any questions. Before you leave the hospital, make certain you can repeat back to the doctor or nurse your diagnosis, any procedures that were done, and your discharge instructions. You also need to know what the plan is for follow-up and when your next appointment is with your doctor. If any consultants saw you in the hospital, you need to know if a follow-up appointment is necessary.

You should have at least a twelve-hour notification of when you are to be discharged. If you require home health visits or other home care, such as equipment, you should get at least twenty-four hours' notice. Do not push your doctor about discharge. A discharge that comes too early increases the risk of a readmission. Doctors are sensitive to repeated requests for discharge, and sometimes a bit too anxious to accommodate their patients, thinking multiple requests for discharge indicate a readiness to take on care at home. Unfortunately, repeated patient demands for discharge are more often indicative of an intense dissatisfaction with the care in the hospital.

If you feel you are not ready, the discharge date can be negotiated with your physician. Doctors and hospitals are being pressured to discharge patients as quickly as possible to reduce costs. Be realistic and have parameters and goals you must achieve for discharge. This could include being able to get out of bed and use the bathroom. If you live alone you should be able to prepare your meals. Remember there are many effective support services to care for you at home including nursing care and IV drug therapy. Your home is a much safer place to receive follow-up care than the hospital with its many errors and dangerous infectious germs.

Your nurse or a hospital social worker can help you make arrangements for your care at home, if you require it. Do not let this go unattended. You want to get home as soon as possible, and it will be very frustrating and possibly expensive for you if the reason you cannot be discharged has to do with the logistics of setting up for your care after discharge. You will need help after surgery for at least a day, and depending on the reason for admission, you will not feel like your normal self for at least a week. In some cases, you may need to transition through a rehabilitation hospital or aftercare residence. This is arranged through your nurse or the hospital social worker. If you can arrange for your aftercare before you are admitted to the hospital, that is a much better alternative.

An in-depth discussion of any tests is best accomplished after the results are available. Some of your test results may not be available until after your discharge. When your test results are back, your doctor or a representative will communicate them to you. You will have a lot of questions, and it is best if at all possible to speak with the doctor who ordered the test. You want to know what question the test was designed to address, was the answer obtained, and what it means for you. Take notes if possible. If not, ask the doctor for either a copy of the results or a written interpretation of the medical report in clear English. Make certain you are able to say back to the doctor what the test results were and what they mean.

You should not leave the hospital unaccompanied. Ask a friend or family member to help you with the discharge process and get settled in your home or the rehab or assisted-care facility where you will continue your recovery.

Few individuals enter medicine or nursing to get rich. The technical terms for these folks are burned out or disappointed. Almost everyone who is in healthcare is seeking the satisfaction and feelings of personal worth that come with doing a job that saves lives and improves the health of their patients. In a way, as a patient you are the agent of that satisfaction. The exercise of courtesy by the staff to you and to each other will go a long way toward increasing the satisfaction your doctors and nurses receive by caring for you. As the glue that keeps the team together, you and your family can be the model of that behavior.

Everything Changes

When we began our careers over forty years ago, the community hospital focused its mission on service to the local community. Patients with complex problems or who required treatment requiring costly equipment were referred to regional hospitals, usually academic medical centers.

The academic centers served patients from their local area, as well as from around the country and even from around the world. Patients were referred because of the expertise and ability of the centers to diagnose and manage difficult medical conditions or rare diseases. The skill and knowledge available at the referral center was the best available at the time, but the academic center often lacked the personal care available at a community hospital. The patient's primary care doctor, the doctor who first recognized a problem or referred the patient for more sophisticated care, no longer remained involved in the patient's care.

In the community hospital, the family doctor directed his patient's care, and since the family doctor was familiar with the special needs and circumstances the patient faced at home, care could be customized to the patient's requirements. The patient and family members often had friends on the hospital or medical staff and the care delivered was not only polite, it was delivered as if the patients were friends or neighbors, which they often were.

Your Doctors' Manners Matter

This has changed dramatically. Hospitals are the centers of multibillion-dollar businesses, employing thousands of workers. The general hospital is gone. Community hospitals have morphed into hospital systems and all patients, from those with commonly occurring illnesses to those with esoteric diseases, are admitted to regional medical centers, often part of a network of hospitals or part of a national corporate hospital chain. The hospital administrator, now called a CEO, earns a salary similar to that of CEOs of large corporations. Some hospitals are organized as profit-generating businesses, others as not-for-profit institutions, but in both cases the CEO seeks to meet the needs of the hospital's patient base, no longer limited to the surrounding community, by providing ever more expensive services and reducing costs in attempts to maximize net income.

How does this work? Academic medical centers continue to train more specialists than they need to staff the central institution. Once their training is completed, these exceptional and highly qualified individuals move into hospitals in the community to establish practices of their own. Community hospitals, eager to limit the number of patients transferred out of their care and eager to attract new types of patients, buy the sophisticated equipment the specialists require. The costs are high, and in order to justify the equipment and to keep the specialists' skills at the cutting edge, hospitals compete aggressively against each other and the academic center for patients both within their community as well as outside their traditional referral area. The result is smaller community hospitals with fewer resources are unable to buy the equipment necessary to attract the specialists. Hospitals lose even those patients who do not require expensive or unusual services. The smaller community hospitals either close or are bought by their larger neighbors. Larger hospitals grow bigger and bigger in size and are ever more sophisticated and expensive to operate.

The challenge is to control costs in highly utilized but low income-generating areas like patient rooms while sophisticated equipment and the highly trained staff needed to operate that equipment sits underutilized. This places great strain on a hospital budget and translates into fewer nurses available to care for patients, more responsibility for the individual nurse, and less satisfaction for the patient and the nurse.

The staff no longer identifies with their patients. The attending physician, usually a hospitalist or a specialist, is not familiar with the patients' social needs. Although most hospital personnel are pleasant and highly competent, they are now caring for patients who live in different communities, the personal connection is lost, and with it the almost reflex response and sensitivity of one neighbor to another.

How does this affect the way you are treated in the hospital? You might point your finger at the obvious.

Your Doctors' Manners Matter

Fewer nurses have less time to spend with each patient and are more likely to be rushed and stressed and appear uncivil. But being polite, offering a trained smile and a reflexive good morning does not take all that much time. Even an extra "pop-in" visit by the nurse to check on a patient only takes an extra three minutes. The real culprit is a corporate philosophy that treats all service people, nurses, doctors, and technicians, as commodities, the idea that one worker can substitute for the other, no one is unique. As the labor force is treated, so are the patients.

The service you receive in your local pharmacy provides a familiar everyday example of how the change in hospital structure affects the care you receive. Back in the day, the pharmacist owned the store, handed you your prescription, and had a personal interest in your care. The pharmacist knew you, knew who was waiting for you at home, knew your kids, and was responsive and considerate of your needs. Today the pharmacy that handles your prescriptions is run by a national chain, you have probably never met the person responsible for making up your order, and even the brief personal interchange with the tech is now disappearing with the rise of mail-order pharmacies.

There are many potential interactions in a hospital setting where the behavior of the personnel makes a critical difference in the quality of the healthcare you receive. Several years ago, one of our patients experienced the new onset of chest pain while driving in his car far from home. He saw a large sign advertising the completion of a new $50 million "center of cardiovascular excellence" in a community medical center close by. He pulled off the road, his wife took the wheel, and they drove to the medical center's emergency department. While his wife parked their car, the patient went to the admissions clerk and told her he had chest pain. At this point, she should have immediately summoned a physician or a triage nurse to determine if the pain was life threatening or if it was safe for him to wait his turn. Instead, the clerk told him to complete his insurance information before the doctor would see him. Following this, he was directed to the waiting area. Anxious and in pain and not yet having had contact with a trained medical professional, he stopped a passing nurse and told her of his chest pain. She repeated the clerk's instructions to wait in the waiting room. Not until the physician examined him, an hour after he walked into the ED, did he receive appropriate care. The delay in receiving care could have resulted in serious and irreparable damage to heart tissue. Damage that could have been prevented.

Fortunately, his pain was not due to a heart attack. When he returned home and came into the office, we informed him of the rule that applies to all hospitals receiving Medicare and Medicaid funds (which effectively means all hospitals): patients with potentially life-threatening conditions must be seen and evaluated immediately and without regard to ability to pay. Our patient wrote a letter of complaint to the hospital administrator. He received a reply from the nurse in charge of the emergency department who wrote to say she was sorry he was not happy with his care. The letter contained no mention or recognition of the hospital's awareness that they had violated important aspects of patient safety and federal law.

Such incidents are not isolated. Another patient, not one of ours, underwent a procedure in the radiology department of a major hospital. While she waited on a gurney in the hallway, the radiologist reviewed the films of her procedure and decided more were needed to complete the studies. The woman was not feeling well. It was time for her medications, and she knew if she did not return to her room immediately they would be given late. She asked the radiology technologist to return her to her room. The tech was under instructions not to release the patient until the radiologist approved the study, and she communicated this to the patient. The woman then asked to speak with the radiologist and explain her concerns, but the doctor replied he was too busy. When the patient did finally return to her room, the nurse repeated her vital signs. Her blood pressure was very high, possibly a result of having missed a dose of her blood pressure lowering pills. She suffered a small stroke that evening.

A patient scheduled for an endoscopy, an examination of her stomach and small intestine by use of a flexible tube inserted into her esophagus, received no food or water overnight as preparation for the procedure. Because of emergencies and scheduling mishaps, the test was delayed several times during the day. By the time the endoscopy laboratory called for her, twenty hours had passed. She received a sedative for the procedure, as is usually done, but because she was slightly dehydrated from almost a full day without nutrition or fluids, her blood pressure was slightly depressed. The sedation lowered her blood pressure further and resulted in a heart attack.

A local hospital advertised on large billboards and TV the top grades they received from a healthcare consulting company for the quality of nursing care on their orthopedic unit. A ninety-year-old patient cared for on that unit required daily ambulation to keep her muscles limber and prevent pressure sores. However, due to a missed communication between the patient's nurse and the physical therapy department, she was not taken out of bed for daily walks down the hallway. The nurse expected physical therapy (PT) to exercise her, and each day PT came to visit, they passed over her because she was sleeping. Because communication between the nurse and PT had been strained ever since the PT tech was cited for unnecessary disruption of a patient's quiet time, the information that the patient did not receive her

Your Doctors' Manners Matter

daily therapy was not passed along to the nurse. The result was a prolonged hospitalization and delayed recovery in a very fragile patient.

Not all hospitals have a bone marrow unit (BMU), but if a hospital wants to be known as a cancer treatment center, such a unit is a necessity. Because of their vulnerability to infection, patients in the BMU are cared for in a special secured area. Each visitor must hand wash for thirty seconds and gown in an entrance room designed for that purpose. A sign, prominently displayed in the room, describes the simple but effective routine. The families understand the importance of this requirement and are very conscientious. However, some hospital personnel resent the extra effort and time required. During one period, a unit experienced an unusual outbreak of infection jeopardizing the lives of several patients. The hospital's infection control team evaluated the outbreak and determined the problem was due to inadequate hand washing precautions. They assigned a secretary to stay in the hand washing room. Her instructions were to observe but not comment. She was just there. The infection rate returned to zero in a very short time.

A rude, inconsiderate admission clerk followed by an inadequate response from the responsible administrator, doctors too busy to speak with their patients, thoughtless care of the patient, poor communication on the ward, and arrogance concerning basic rules of infection control. At first glance, you might think there is little you or your family can do to remedy these situations.

No! You will not put up with rude behavior from your children. If a sales clerk is rude you will probably not return to the store. If a co-worker is rude you might calmly express your concerns with him or her in private, and failing that, if your work is affected, you might ask your supervisor to intervene.

We believe most instances of inappropriate or rude behavior arise not out of evil-intentioned individuals but are the result of personnel who have temporarily lost their focus because they are rushed, stressed, overworked, or tired. A gentle reminder is sometimes all that is needed. A firm refusal to engage the offender in a debate may be necessary. To impose punishment on an individual for rudeness, other than social isolation and an occasional imperious glance, is itself wrong and violates the precepts of good manners. You are not the manners vigilante. As Miss Manners states:

> What, then, does one do with one's justified anger? Miss Manners' meager arsenal consists only of the withering look, the insistent and repeated request, the cold voice, the report up the chain of command and the tilted nose. They generally work. When they fail, she has the ability to dismiss inferior behavior from her mind as coming from inferior people.

Your Doctors' Manners Matter

In the hospital, good manners are not just about agreeable behavior demonstrating respect. As we discussed in previous chapters, good manners are essential to providing good care. Let someone know if you feel you are not receiving proper attention and that may include asking to see a physician or supervising nurse. If that does not work, ask a friend or family member or your clergyman, if necessary, to intervene for you at the administrative level.

The Joint Commission (TJC, formerly known as JCAHO) is a voluntary not-for-profit organization that accredits all member healthcare institutions in the US. A hospital must be a member of the TJC to qualify for Medicare and Medicaid funds. The organization provides onsite inspections of hospitals and outpatient facilities and is responsible for determining if the organization is in compliance with the Medicare standards of quality performance. According to the mission statement, TJC strives to "continuously improve healthcare for the public…"[1] The manual runs to thousands of pages of requirements, visits can be announced or unannounced, and should a hospital fail its inspection, it can be put on probation and if necessary, operations can be shut down.

In January 2009, TJC issued standards that addressed disruptive and inappropriate behavior in healthcare institutions, behavior that can result in poor medical outcomes. These standards encourage hospitals to adopt a code of conduct to define "acceptable and disruptive and inappropriate behaviors" and "educate all team members—both physician and non-physician staff—on appropriate professional behavior defined by the organization's code of conduct. The code and education should emphasize respect [and] include training in basic business etiquette and people skills."[2] The remainder of the document mentions desirable behaviors only once and disruptive, unprofessional, or intimidating behavior fifteen times. Although some forms of undesirable behavior are spelled out, such as violence and criminal acts, other undesirable behaviors fall under the category of "I know it when I see it," such as condescending language or voice intonation (any married couple will immediately recognize the difficulty).

Unfortunately, the definition of acceptable behavior and of inappropriate and disruptive behavior can be subjective. The good news is that TJC alert on behavior instructs hospitals to adopt a code of conduct that emphasizes respect. If the staff shows respect to each other and their patients, they are halfway toward displaying good manners, for as we have argued, the display of good manners is a way of showing respect.

Good manners cannot be legislated. Good manners arise from the desire of the individual to conform to behavior the local society considers beneficial to its survival. The local society can be the neighborhood, the town, or the working community. The desire to conform is a result of a wish to succeed, or to be liked or respected, or just to be considered a valuable member of the group.

The practice of good manners should be encouraged. Failure to make the effort to appear agreeable in stressful situations results in churlishness, verbal outbursts, passive-aggressive behavior, and plain old rudeness.§§ We all have a moral obligation to be agreeable. As we and others have pointed out, rude behavior indicates a lack of moral character. More importantly, acting in a manner that appears to indicate respect for others can inspire individuals to actually consider the dignity of others. The special pleasure we receive when treated in a moral way inspires similar treatment to others. So rather than legislating interpersonal behavior in the hospital and clinic, we modestly propose encouraging good manners and appropriate behavior. We suggest that such behavior will encourage similar behavior among colleagues and patients. Rather than staff seeking out transgressors and villains and reporting to whatever group accepts such reports (Human Resources is the usual suspect), we suggest a manners squad giving instruction to those who demonstrate a need to know how to act in given situations.

---

§§ It is also an inefficient way to get results, what with having to deal with angry personnel and frequently with tears in addition to whatever it was that resulted in the outburst in the first place.

Of course, egregious behavior that "undermines a culture of safety" must be eliminated.*** In today's complex medical world, it is all about teamwork. The doctor tells the following story.

* * *

Dr. Robert J. is a dedicated, concerned physician who places the welfare of his patients before his own comfort. He is an internist, respected by his colleagues and the nurses he works with, and loved by his patients for his caring manner and responsiveness. If he has one fault, it is that he asks everyone he works with for the same commitment to his patients and becomes visibly annoyed when he believes that commitment is not forthcoming.

Central Regional Medical Center, established in 1970 to serve its mostly suburban community as a 200-bed general hospital, has been a success story. As the local population grew, so did the not-for-profit institution. CRMC built or acquired a number of outpatient clinics and surgery centers in surrounding communities and bought two additional hospitals. The original building has been added on to and is now an 800-bed general hospital. The two smaller institutions, both general

---

*** Although several AMA and TJC reports and publications do list all manners of outlawed behavior—foul language, threatening language, facial expressions, and (bad) manners—it would be impossible to list all forms of obnoxious behavior. And in any event, the judgment that the behavior interfered with care can be subjective at best or retaliatory or even fabricated.

medical and surgical hospitals, serve the surrounding rural areas.

Dr. J. has staff privileges at the main hospital, but admits the majority of his patients to the rural hospital, Western Community Medical Center. One Sunday evening as he sat down to supper with his wife and all three teenage children, a rare weekend event, Dr. J. received a page from his answering service to call Joy Williams, a patient he had been following for several weeks with symptoms of intermittent headache, weight loss, and palpitations. He has known her for fifteen years, ever since she first came to him for her college physical.

Joy married when she was twenty-five, enjoyed good health until recently, and bore two children without difficulty. She recently returned to the work force as a public relations vice president for a locally based national food company. This is how Dr. J. tells the story:

"When I returned the page, her husband answered the phone. It was clear he was struggling to control his voice.

'Joy's not acting right,' he said.

'What do you mean?' I asked.

'Well, when we got home from the lake, she said she had a headache. I told her to take a nap, that I would fix dinner. She went into the bedroom, but came out in her nightie and slippers and said she was late for the office.'

'What then?'

'I took away her car keys, of course.' He chuckled, but I knew he was trying to minimize his fear.

'We had a fight. She cried, went to bed, and then came out five minutes later and asked for the dog. She had a weird look in her eyes and kept searching about. The dog died a year ago.'"

Dr. J. continues his story. "When I saw Joy in the office the previous week, her blood pressure was mildly elevated, and I was trying to decide if I should admit her for a workup or try to do it as an outpatient. I knew if I admitted her I would have a tough time justifying it to the insurance company, but doing the workup as an outpatient would take so long, and the possibilities for screw up, especially on the twenty-four-hour urine collection I wanted to order, were infinite. Now I had something to tell the insurance company, but I hated that I had delayed until she had such severe symptoms.

"I told her husband we would admit her to Western, and that I would be over as soon as she was admitted. I have all the numbers of the two CRMC hospitals in my cellphone contacts list, so I called the admissions desk on my cellphone. I told admissions to expect her, left some routine orders, and asked for the nurse to call me when my patient settled into her room. I planned to order routine blood and chemistry work, and get the twenty-four-hour urine collection started. If they were abnormal, we could do the MRI studies late the next day or Tuesday at the latest. I was more certain than ever that we were dealing with a tumor, and I needed to prove it quickly so we could get the woman operated on before she got worse, even died. So I was feeling pressed and a little guilty that I had waited. Not that I am excusing my following behavior, just trying to explain it.

"I waited and waited and no call. It was about eleven. So, I called Mr. Williams back on his cell phone and asked what had happened. He said he was waiting to speak with me at the bedside. That they had gotten settled by eight. Three hours. I was pissed. Why hadn't the nurse called? What about my instructions? Now it would be impossible to get the urine collection done in time to get the MRI the next day; we would have to wait for Tuesday morning. She could have a seizure by then. And on top of that, the nurse hadn't even called me with the vital signs. Joy's blood pressure was definitely an issue, and I was sure her husband thought I didn't care enough to hustle over to meet him.

"When I got to the hospital I checked the computer. Joy had been admitted to the third floor at 7:48. I went directly to her room. She was asleep. I asked Mr. Williams if there was any change since he spoke with me, and he said no. Then he told me the nurse had been waiting for my call so I could give her admission orders. Waiting for my call? I had asked her to call me.

"I reassured Mr. Williams that we would start the testing immediately, and then I stormed over to the nurses' station. Of course the nurse, a young woman I think was working for maybe three months, they always put the newbies on at night, looked up, smiled, and said 'Good evening, Dr. J.'

"Now, I am not proud of what followed. I only offer it as a cautionary tale. I have certainly learned a lesson. At first, I ignored her and picked up Mrs. Williams chart to review her vital signs. Her BP was high, 140/110. I needed to treat that right away, but not so high I was afraid she would die. Her pulse was 100, also high. I put down the chart and leaned over the nurse's desk.

'Why didn't you call me like I asked?' I said. Her smile faded and she suddenly looked a little sick. Even now I feel badly about how I behaved. 'I called the admissions desk and left a message for the admitting nurse to call me.' My voice was getting louder and louder, and I am sure I looked angry.

'I didn't get any message from admissions. Mr. Williams said you would be in. The patient just showed up, no orders, so I put her to bed.'

'Oh really. You're saying I didn't leave a message or orders?'

"So this is my first mistake. I should have just let it go, chalked it up as a screw-up. After all, they happen every day, and on the grand scale of things, this was not a very important one at that. No one died. Instead, I put words in the young woman's mouth. As if to say she was calling me a liar. What was I thinking? That she had made an error and my berating her would prevent any future errors? That if I made her feel badly enough, she would never again make any mistakes?

"Just then the nurse supervisor, Miss Wallace, happened along. She smiled. Looked from me to the nurse and back. Saw my anger and that her nurse was near tears. 'What's the problem?' she asked.

"I explained about my calls. Having to wait. Missing an opportunity. That the nurse was accusing me of practically abandoning my patient.

'I can prove I left a message.' I dialed the admissions clerk on the hospital phone, a woman I know by first name. My hand was shaking, I was so angry. 'Cheryl, this is Dr. J. I have Miss Wallace up here. Tell her the message I gave you when I called in the admission.'

'You never called in an admission, Dr. J. Sorry. Your patient just showed up.'

"Miss Wallace and the nurse must have heard. They were staring daggers at me. Wallace's lips were so tight they looked glued together. She and I have never been friendly, and I could almost hear her complaining to the CEO.

'Now come on. We spoke. It was about seven. You must have come on duty just before.'

'You never spoke with me.'

"At this point I was getting paranoid. I was thinking for some reason Wallace organized a campaign to drive me nuts, and it was working. I took a deep breath, trying to figure out what the hell was going on. That's the only thing that saved me from erupting, trying to noodle out the problem. I know Cheryl. She would not lie to me. Something was terribly wrong.

'I'm going to get to the bottom of this tomorrow,' I told them. 'But for now, just take the orders and see if you can get something done tonight.' Again, I couldn't help myself. Sarcasm never works. No one appreciates it as a joke and everyone in hearing distance is insulted when it's meant as a putdown. I was fuming, but I wrote the orders in a steady hand. Miss Wallace told the young nurse to leave and get herself together, that she would deal with the orders, and in fact, she did get the tests going.

"First, as far as the patient was concerned, I put her on meds to bring down her BP. Her urine test was positive. She did have a tumor, a pheochromocytoma, on MRI. The slight delay in diagnosis was nothing compared to trying to get OR time. But we got it done, and Joy Williams is fine.

"Marianne Wallace did in fact report me to the CEO, who filed a complaint with the Medical Executive Committee. They asked me to explain my actions. By that time, I had figured out what had happened. I checked my cell phone records the next day and discovered I had called the main CRMC hospital admissions clerk rather than the clerk at Western. The woman I spoke with had in fact taken the message, and as far as I know is still waiting for the Williams family to show. As Cheryl said, I never spoke with her.

"I apologized to the nurse that day, and she graciously accepted my apology. She excused my rude behavior and laid it off to the hour and my desire to get started on a treatment plan for my patient. I also apologized to Miss Wallace, and although she frostily accepted my apology, both oral and written, the fact is she reported me.

"This could all have been avoided if I had first assumed that everyone was doing their job as best they could, and some other explanation other than an intense desire to obstruct my plans was the cause of the delay. Second, I could have accepted what the nurse said and not responded to it, even if I did not believe her. After all, if she were lying about not receiving my message, how would calling her attention to it change her behavior? And last, losing my temper served no earthly purpose. It did not make me feel better, it made everyone around me feel awful, it slowed down the process of getting my patient cared for, and I could have potentially ruined a young nurse's career."

* * *

Dr. J. learned from his aggressive behavior, but the lesson was hard won. Many doctors demonstrate rude behavior, many nurses display passive-aggressive behavior, and many administrators disrespect both doctors and nurses and rule with an autocratic hand. It is a war out there, and when a battle is occurring whether in the OR, hospital ward, or administrative office, you, the patient, are the battlefield and suffer the most from these conflicts. You may feel your surgeon is an unapproachable, god-like figure, worshipped by his office staff, the ultimate caregiver, but if that worship is not coupled with respect and really good communication your healthcare will suffer even in the hands of the most skillful.

How much easier would it have been on everyone if previously Dr. J. had been offered instruction on proper behavior under stressful situations? He knew he had an obsessive personality. The risk that he would offend a co-worker was high. Dr. J. wanted to act in an appropriate manner. He knows how important it is to act in an agreeable manner for his colleagues to want to work with him. That appropriate behavior issues forth not from rules and regulations, but from an inner desire to act agreeably is not a new idea.

Your Doctors' Manners Matter

We will all do a lot better if we know how our good behavior will further the goal of improving our health, and if we see the results in action. To exact revenge for a real or imagined transgression results in two instances of rude behavior. In some situations, the only good example available to the healthcare team is a gracious patient.

Chapter Five
The Hospital Experience
Issues Addressed in this Chapter

- When you are a patient in the hospital, you are a member of the healthcare team.
- When you enter the emergency department, a professional member of the medical team should quickly evaluate your complaint.
- Many hospitals use hospitalists rather than personal physicians to care for patients.
- One doctor should be in charge of coordinating your care while you are in the hospital.
- Everyone who cares for you should introduce himself or herself and state their role.
- If you have a problem you cannot resolve, the patient representative can help.
- Your primary care nurse is the nurse who will help you navigate your way through the hospital.
- The Joint Commission Hospital Standards encourages hospitals to adopt a code of conduct to educate healthcare workers on appropriate behavior.
- When you leave the hospital, you will receive clearly written instructions to continue your care at home.

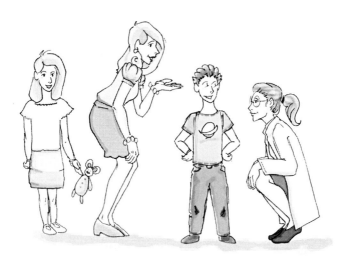

Chapter Six

At the Pediatrician: A Teachable Moment

A person's a person, no matter how small.

– Dr. Seuss

The pediatrician provides healthcare to prevent and treat illness in children. Your child might see the same pediatrician from birth through the adolescent years. Where the pediatricians' practices differ from those of the adult medical specialists is in the special challenges and opportunities that come with caring for the newborn, child, preadolescent, and adolescent. Most adults between the ages of twenty and fifty never visit the doctor's office except for an acute illness, such as a fever or cold or the new onset of pain. The well-child visit, on the other hand, is an important part of maintaining a child's health, and includes immunizations, first year of life visits, and physical exams to check for normal growth and development, physical exams for school and participation in sports.

Are You Talking to Me?

A special challenge for you as the parent is how to best balance your natural role as the complete caregiver with the professional responsibility the doctor has to care for the medical needs of the child. In the first years of life, your child is totally dependent on you for healthcare. During this period, the conversation in the medical office is between you and the doctor. As your child grows and matures, the doctor can spend time speaking with your child. For the very young child, this will mostly be social conversation, or play. In the case of the older child, the doctor may question your child directly to bring out signs and symptoms of disease. During the part of the consultation when you and your doctor are discussing how to approach treatment, if any is needed, very little of the conversation will include the young child.

As your child gets older, he or she can contribute more information about symptoms and the course of any illness. Your child will also cooperate more fully with the exam process. Although the doctor might engage the older child more often during the socialization and exam process of the consultation, it is just as important to include the older child and adolescent in conversations concerning the diagnosis and any recommendations for treatment. The wise pediatrician and parent recognize that an older child is competent to participate in at least some of that conversation, often showing insight into school and daily routines that influence treatment regimens. Older children might wish to raise concerns about routines that may not be compatible with their schedule or social life. While you may still feel completely responsible and therefore try to maintain control over the details of your child's treatment, with the older child, preadolescent and adolescent, control of the treatment regimen falls increasingly into your child's hands. The doctor should therefore enlist your child into any discussions about treatment options. Children over the age of seven, in general, can give information about their symptoms and also help in figuring out the best way to approach their treatment. Many adolescents can coordinate their own care, with little parental supervision.

Including your child in discussions and decision making about any illness has an added benefit. This is an opportunity for your child to have an adult interaction in a safe and controlled atmosphere. This will provide experience and foster confidence in the ability to relate to an adult during a conversation about an important subject—in this case, his or her health. Children can participate actively in their healthcare, and when included in the treatment plans, will engage and cooperate to a greater extent with the plan.

Look for a pediatrician who can communicate well with your child in an age-appropriate manner. With the younger child, your pediatrician should know how to put him or her at ease by making the physical exam a sort of playtime. With the older child, your pediatrician should encourage conversation. In many cultures, children are expected to remain silent in the company of adults, and in this situation parents may answer for the child or interrupt a conversation between the doctor and the child. Here the doctor must and should intervene to draw your child into the conversation. You may feel the doctor is not showing respect for your authority, or that your child is not ready to take on responsibility for his or her health; however, by bringing your child into the conversation, the doctor will not only gain your child's confidence and trust, but a successful interaction is an opportunity to learn polite adult behavior, increase confidence, and demonstrate maturity. Most pediatricians will include the preteen and teen in the question-and-answer part of the exam. This is a good opportunity for your child to learn to participate in turn-taking during a conversation. As with the adult patient, the doctor should always show respect for both you and your child by listening carefully, being attentive to your needs, and making certain all your questions are answered.

As a parent, you may feel guilt or anxieties concerning the origins of your child's illness. Many parents are reluctant to raise these fears, and your doctor, with some discretion, must address them in order to arrive at a practical course of treatment. Otherwise you might believe one possible source of the problem was not considered, and you might be tempted to seek another doctor's diagnosis and opinion. It is therefore important that you raise these concerns with your child's doctor before you leave the office.

The unasked question almost always produces more anxiety than the answer. Ask the question. Say something like "How did my baby get this?" Or more directly, "Is there anything I/we did that caused this?" Your doctor will address the question honestly, and you can move on. The need to know why your child is ill is one of the important goals of any medical consultation.

In the exam room, when the doctor is talking with your child and especially when the doctor is explaining a treatment plan, try not to be distracted by your child or siblings. Take notes. Repeat back to the doctor any point you may find confusing. Ask the doctor to repeat the plan. If you believe your child did not understand, ask him or her.

Before leaving the doctor's office, you and your child should be in agreement with the doctor as to what the problem is, what caused it, and how to deal with it. You should be able to "say back" to the doctor the diagnosis, the treatment, and the plans for follow-up.

Caring for the Teenager

We know of young adults in their twenties, lifelong patients of their pediatricians, who become quite upset when told they will be referred to an internist because of their age. On the other hand, some teens refuse to visit the same pediatrician as their younger siblings, finding a doctor's office that caters to infants and toddlers and decorated with cartoon characters too juvenile for their sensibilities.

The best doctor for your teen is one who has a long-standing relationship with him or her. However families move, doctors retire or relocate, or your pediatrician's offices do not treat teens. There is a subspecialty of pediatrics that deals with the problems of teenagers called adolescent medicine. If you are looking for a doctor for your teen, be sure and ask when you call the pediatrician's office if they treat teens, and if they have a board certified or board qualified adolescent medicine specialist on staff. Some internists have taken a certification exam in adolescent medicine and can provide excellent care for your teen as well.

Seek out a doctor who has the ability to establish a trusting relationship, shows respect for your teen by exhibiting those characteristics we discussed in Chapter Three, and can communicate openly with him or her. Your teen will respond positively toward a doctor who can talk openly with him or her in a safe and comfortable office environment and in an unhurried manner. Of particular importance to most teens is to find a pediatrician of the same sex. Some teens respond better to an older doctor, some to a younger doctor. You know your child, but it's a tough guess as to the age, looks, and dress of the doctor your teen will be most comfortable with. The most important characteristic is how well the doctor communicates with your teen, and you should ask your teen and the doctor after the first visit how they thought the visit progressed.

Some teens may prefer to speak with the doctor without the parent in the room. The teen may state this desire spontaneously, or your doctor may ask if he or she would like the opportunity to speak with the doctor alone or to be examined in private. A same-sex chaperone during a physical exam with a teenager is always advisable and is mandatory if the physician is of the opposite sex.

A private exam with the doctor is an opportunity for the child to discuss issues they believe will result in either increased tension or outright confrontation with their adult guardian or parent. Some parents balk at this, believing they have been frozen out of a conversation they have every right to be part of. The only alternative to not cooperating with your child's request for private time with the doctor is not giving your child the opportunity to discuss a bothersome issue with an expert. More often than not, after the private consultation, the pediatrician will ask the teen if he or she would like to bring the adult into the conversation, if appropriate. As with guilt, it's the unanswered questions that engender the most anxiety.

What You Can Do

As the guardian of your child's health and the intermediary between your child and the doctor, there are several steps you can take to ensure the success of the visit to the pediatrician. First, never use the doctor as a threatened punishment. When we run our errands around town, we sometimes hear parents threaten misbehaving children with a trip to the doctor, or that the doctor will give the misbehaving child a shot. This is inappropriate and will make for a very unpleasant time of it at the next doctor visit. Most pediatricians' offices are arranged in a manner that will appeal to children of

Your Doctors' Manners Matter

various ages in an attempt to make the visit to the doctor an enjoyable experience. Negative comments and threats will undermine this important endeavor.

When making a well-child appointment, try to block out a full morning or afternoon. Pediatricians are often delayed by emergencies, harried parents' phone calls, and unscheduled trips to the hospital or emergency department to see a patient. If you are rushed or otherwise upset by a delay in the office, the young child will feel the anxiety and tend to reflect it in their behavior. The first appointment in the morning is your best bet for the doctor to be close to on time.

If possible, do not wait for the weekend or late evening to make a call for a sick-child visit. These visits are much easier to schedule when made earlier in the day and the outcome of the visit will be more efficient and possibly end with a better result than a trip to an emergency department or walk-in clinic and a visit with doctors unfamiliar with your family. Of course, not all emergencies come during the day. Many pediatricians are members of a group or have consolidated a number of groups to operate an off-hours phone system. Also, some practices conduct evening and weekend hours for working families and can fit a sick-child visit into those appointments.

Keep your own record of the immunizations and medications your child receives. The American Academy of Pediatrics publication, *Your Child's Health Record,* is available to order singly for about $4.00.[1] Many pediatricians' offices will supply you with that or a similar form to keep for your records. One form from the CDC is available on the Internet for download at www.immunize.org/catg.d/p2022.pdf. Taking such a form with you whenever you visit a doctor for your child's care will simplify and improve the results of the visit.

Immunizations

After maintaining proper nutrition and hygiene, keeping your child's immunization record up-to-date is the single most important medical task you can accomplish to prevent serious illness. How effective are immunizations? Smallpox, once a scourge that killed 30 percent of those infected, and in the nineteenth century killed up to 10 percent of babies in the first year of life, has been eliminated from the human population. Polio, one of the most dreaded childhood diseases of the twentieth century in the United States, caused epidemics throughout the nineteenth and twentieth century, up until the introduction of the Salk inactivated poliovirus vaccine (IPV) in 1956. An average of over 35,000 cases/year were reported during this time period, and then in 1957, the first full year of widespread campaigns to immunize children against polio, the number of cases rapidly declined to under 2,500. By 1965, only sixty-one cases of paralytic polio were reported.[2]

Your Doctors' Manners Matter

However, with the exception of smallpox, the viruses and bacteria that cause childhood diseases persist in the unimmunized or inadequately immunized population.

Recent small-scale outbreaks of measles, whooping cough, and other childhood diseases highlight in bold strokes the importance of childhood immunizations. Outbreaks only occur in communities with unimmunized children, even if the percent of unimmunized children is small. Deliberately withholding immunization from your child does not give him or her an advantage over the other children. Just the opposite. It puts your child at serious risk for life-threatening disease.

Unfortunately, newborn babies are not fully protected until six months old, even when their immunizations are current. Those parents who choose not to immunize their children not only put their own child at risk, they put the most helpless, newborn babies, at risk as well. Adults, especially those who have contact with young infants, are advised to get the adult version of the tetanus, diphtheria, pertussis vaccine (Tdap) as their booster shot.

An inexpensive way to obtain needed childhood immunizations is through a public health clinic. If you use a public health clinic, keep your child's immunization record up-to-date and show your doctor the record when you keep your appointments for the well-baby exams.

Silverman, MD and Adler, MD

What to Look for When You are Looking for a Pediatrician

Ease of scheduling is important to a busy parent if you have a sick child. When you call the pediatrician's office, there should be an easy way of talking to a real person, preferably a physician's assistant or experienced nurse. Most pediatricians will have a period of time blocked out for sick-child visits. Some offices are open on off business hours so working parents can take their well child for a checkup without missing work. This is an important courtesy that marks a practice sympathetic to patients and families. Some offices arrange for counseling sessions after regular hours. A busy pediatrician cannot address the complex issues involved with bed wetting, eating disorders, truancy, obstinacy, etc. in the ten or fifteen minutes allotted for a patient visit. Offices with these non-traditional scheduling plans demonstrate a responsibility to the patient and respect for parents trying to juggle multiple responsibilities.

When you first walk into the pediatricians' office, you can get an idea about how thoughtful the doctors are in their approach to their patients by the interior design and decoration of the office and how it differs from that of the adult specialist. The office should be inviting. The interior of the office should be well lit and the waiting room decorated in bright colors and murals. An office with one or two unique activities or displays will mean children will look forward to their visit. One pediatrician we heard about is a model train hobbyist. A large-scale train set runs through his office and into different rooms. Many pediatricians have one or two (quiet) games of skill such as might be found in an arcade. Another has a large aviary. Even a large fish tank can be of interest, although live animals require regular maintenance.

The exam rooms might each be decorated and named for a theme: the princess room, the comic book character room, the jungle room, the superhero room, etc. At least one exam room should be tailored to the older child or adolescent who might not appreciate a physical exam in a room dominated by talking mice and ducks.

Careful attention in design should be given to reduce transmission of contagious diseases. One waiting area should be reserved for sick-child visits, that is for children with colds or fevers. Alternatively, ill children should be ushered immediately into an exam room. Parents with upper respiratory complaints or coughs should be encouraged to reschedule their well child's appointment rather than accompany them to the office. Alcohol scrub and sink stations should be placed liberally around the office and in the exam rooms. The toys available to the children should be both age appropriate and completely washable. In the sick room, once used they should be removed for the day and washed and never shared. Chairs should be comfortable and appropriately sized for children and adults. TVs showing age-appropriate shows are great child pleasers in the medical office, although most pediatricians will advise limiting your child's exposure to TV at home. Books may seem like a good idea, but they are impossible to clean. Bring your own books to the office so you can read to your child or so older children can read to themselves. Charging stations are a new idea being adopted by some practices for MP3 players, tablets, and handheld electronic game consoles.

In the Hospital

Many primary care physicians, including pediatricians, prefer to leave the care of hospitalized patients to the hospitalist and emergency department physicians and no longer see patients in the emergency department or in the hospital. We discussed the role of the hospitalist in Chapter Five. An exception is the well newborn baby. In some hospitals, all the well-baby care is done by the doctors who specialize in caring for the sick newborn, the neonatologists. Some pediatricians responsible for following the baby after discharge prefer to establish a relationship with the family soon after the baby's birth.

No matter who provides care for your well baby, ill newborn, or hospitalized child, insist on a copy of the medical summary of your child's stay in the hospital when you leave. If one is not ready, ask for a copy of what is called the "face sheet." This will have the diagnosis listed on it. Also, ask for a copy of the last three days' worth of medical notes. If you are taking home your healthy newborn baby, ask for a copy of the well-baby record. Copies of these records are rightfully yours, although you may have to pay a small copying fee for them. Take these records to your pediatrician on your first office visit. Do not rely on the hospital record room to forward the records to the pediatrician's office. Let us repeat that. *Never rely on the hospital to forward your records to your physician.* Records, even electronic records, have a remarkable ability to get lost in cyberspace, in the medical records department, or in the pediatrician's office. Hand carry the records to your pediatrician. He or she will scan them into the chart. No records lost.

In our experience, those doctors who practice general pediatrics truly believe their patient's health is their first priority. Pediatricians are among the most accessible and dedicated of our colleagues. In the movies, the pediatrician is often portrayed as a kindly dedicated physician. Our experience in working with our colleagues bears out that perception.

Chapter Six
At the Pediatrician: A Teachable Moment
Issues Addressed in this Chapter

- The pediatrician is your first contact for illness in your child and provides follow-up care and regular child screening exams.
- The well-child visit is an important part of maintaining your child's health.
- Older children can be encouraged to contribute to discussions about their illness and their management.
- Look for a pediatrician who can communicate with your child.
- The medical encounter can be an opportunity for a child to learn how to participate in adult style interactions.
- Some teenagers will prefer alone time with the doctor during the exam.

Conclusion

Some Parting Advice

When people talk, listen completely. Most people never listen.

– Ernest Hemingway

As we pointed out in Section One, for some doctors, despite adherence to the ethical principles of medical care, good manners in their professional lives have succumbed to baser standards of popular culture just as they have in private life. While the worst that can happen in the commercial world, if you are confronted with bad manners, is that you will not visit a particular shop or restaurant again, a lapse of manners in the doctor's office can be detrimental to your health.

With the introduction of the Affordable Care Act, many hospitals and doctors' offices have instituted patient satisfaction surveys. Compensation to hospitals can be affected by your response to these questionnaires. Any score less than excellent is noted and addressed. We have noticed that those medical facilities taking the surveys seriously generally receive better scores on non-medical items, such as friendliness of staff, greetings, admission desk function, etc. In the future, doctors and hospitals will also receive additional reimbursement when they meet certain basic guidelines for patient care.

Once You Have Made Your Appointment, How Should You Prepare for Your Visit?

Create a timeline of your complaint. When did the symptom start? Where is it located? When is it most bothersome and when less? What have you done to make it better? Did it help? Make it worse? Make a list of all the hospitalizations you have had. If it's more than five, list those for the last five years. List all the surgeries. You need dates, doctors, reason for the admissions, and positive and negative tests. Chances are you will not be able to remember all the information. This is not a big problem, but more is better. Make a list of all the medications you are on right now—both the name and dose. Include all non-prescription medication as well.

If your visit is to an emergency department, try to go with a friend or family member who is familiar with your problem. Often the anxiety associated with an ED visit can limit a person's ability to tell a full story, and a friend or family member can fill in the missing parts.

When you are speaking with the doctor, feel free to ask questions, take the time to tell your full story, and take notes. Before you leave the doctor's office, be able to repeat the diagnosis and the doctor's instructions. Be clear about any needed follow-up visit. Have a written list of any tests or medications you are supposed to take. If you do not get a printed sheet, take a few minutes and write down the instructions.

Your Doctors' Manners Matter

Other Practical Steps to Take

Try to make your appointment the first one in the morning or after lunch. Do not schedule any time-related obligations for the half-day of your visit. Even a quick follow-up visit can take up to one and a half hours.

Dress appropriately: easy-to-remove clothes, no perfumes or colognes, and keep in mind that most offices will be cool to cold, even in summer.

Show up on time or fifteen minutes early. Turn off your cell phone in the waiting area. Take along something interesting to read, or if you are with your child, playthings. If your visit is to the pediatrician's office, try to find someone to watch the siblings. Consider the day and time. For example, if you are sick on Thursday afternoon, do not wait until Friday night to call the doctor.

Use the emergency departments judiciously. Emergency department visits cost more, wait times are usually longer, and in most cases, you will be asked to see your primary care doctor or a specialist during regular office hours for a timely follow-up. You are saving neither money nor time.

However, if you do have an emergency, then do not hesitate to visit the ED or call an ambulance. What is an emergency? A partial list is: trouble breathing; a child with high fever who is not acting like themselves; a new seizure; severe pain; uncontrolled bleeding; altered level of consciousness; electrical burns; sudden severe headache; head injury with loss of consciousness; vomiting that is uncontrollable, especially if associated with copious watery diarrhea; if you think you have broken a bone, especially if the limb is deformed; chest pain, especially if the pain travels to your left arm or neck or chin or abdomen; if you have suffered serious trauma; for a poison or chemical ingestion (call poison control first); or if someone in your immediate vicinity yells out "call 911!" These are all good reasons, among others, to seek immediate medical attention.

Observing the Observer

In this book we have tried to show how, as a patient, you can assess the abilities of the doctors you see in the office, emergency department, and in the hospital.

In Chapters One through Three, we have shown that good manners in the doctor's office and in the hospital are not just a question of conforming to social norms. Good manners demonstrate a moral commitment to you, your health, and to medicine as a profession. The doctor who makes that commitment will also be the doctor who maintains his level of knowledge by keeping up with the medical literature, attending medical seminars, and a doctor who constantly updates his medical skills and knowledge.

In Chapters Four through Six, we have shown how you can tell if your welfare is more than just a job to the doctors and staff who care for you. When your doctor displays good medical manners by listening to your story and addressing your concerns rather than minimizing them, when your consultation is a two-way street, and when your doctor and the medical staff pay attention to and make necessary accommodations for your special circumstances, you will know you are in good hands. You do not need an advanced degree to know when you are being treated with respect.

* * *

Throughout the consultation, consider the quotation at the beginning of this book. Observe your doctor. Are you treated with respect? Have you been able to tell your story? Have your fears been addressed? Do you feel comfortable when you leave that your doctor is one of those physicians who believes that to take care of you the doctor has to care for you? If so, then you have found the "A-list" doctor. And here is a secret. The A-list doctors tend to socialize with one another and refer to one another. Once you are plugged into the A-list, chances are all your referrals will be on the A-list too.

Most of the doctors we have met in our professional and personal lives have dedicated their practices to their patients' well-being. Among the doctors we trained with, very few decided on medicine as a career because it was a way to make a lot of money. We suspect those who did were greatly disappointed. As the business of medicine changed over the last thirty to forty years, doctors were forced to adopt better business practices, such as less charity care, stricter accounts receivable policies, fewer write-offs, and more selective choices about being on insurance company rosters. Despite these changes to their businesses, doctors continue to adhere to the medical principles that patients come first and that compassion, respect, and professionalism are important attributes of good medical care.

References

Introduction

[1] Austin Flint, *Medical Ethics and Etiquette* (New York: D. Appleton and Company, 1883).
[2] Atul Gawande, *The Checklist Manifesto: How to Get Things Right* (New York: Henry Holt and Company, 2009).
[3] Pauline Chen, "The Hidden Curriculum of Medicine," *The New York Times*, 2009.
[4] Kenneth M. Ludmerer, *Learning to Heal: The Development of American Medical Education* (Baltimore: The Johns Hopkins University Press, 1985).
[5] Diane Payne, "Crisis in Medicine," *Newsweek*, August 22, 2005.
[6] Judith Martin, "A Philosophy in Etiquette," Proceedings of the American Philosophical Society 137, no. 3 (1993).

Chapter One

[1] Kathleen Collins, Ann Duffett, Jean Johnson, and Steve Farkas, "Aggravating Circumstances: A Status Report on Rudeness in America." Public Agenda Foundation, April 2002.

2 Judith Martin, *Miss Manners Rescues Civilization from Sexual Harassment, Frivolous Lawsuits, Dissing and Other Lapses in Civility* (New York: Crown Publishers, 1996).

3 "Women Entering Med School Declining Since Peak Enrollment in 2003," AMA MedEd Update, http://www.ama-assn.org/ama/pub/meded/2012-may/2012-may-top_stories3.shtml. Accessed Mar 3, 2013.

4 "Disputes between Medical Supervisors and Trainees," *Journal of the American Medical Association* 272 (1994): 1861–65.

5 Hippocrates and Galen, *The Writings of Hippocrates and Galen: Of Decency in Manners and In Dress,* trans. John Redman Coxe (Philadelphia: Lindsay & Blakiston, 1846), 74–79.

6 Albert R. Jonsen, *A Short History of Medical Ethics* (New York: Oxford University Press, 2000), 1–12.

7 John Gregory, *Lectures on the Duties and Qualifications of a Physician* (London: W. Strahan and T. Cadell, 1772).

8 Chauncey D. Leake, *Percival's Medical Ethics* (Huntington, New York: Robert E. Krieger, 1975).

9 Robert Baker, Arthur Caplan, Linda Emanuel, and Stephen Latham, *The American Medical Ethics Revolution: How the AMA's Code of Ethics has Transformed Physicians' Relationships to Patients,*

Professionals, and Society (Baltimore: The Johns Hopkins University Press, 1999).

[10] American Medical Association, "Code of Ethics," http://www.ama-assn.org/ama/pub/physician-resources/medical-ethics/code-medical-ethics.page?

[11] Abraham Flexner, *Medical Education: A Comparative Study* (New York: The MacMillan Co., 1925).

[12] Judith Martin, *Common Courtesy: In Which Miss Manners Solves the Problem that Baffled Mr. Jefferson* (New York: Atheneum Press, 1985).

Chapter Two

[1] Philip Tumulty, "What is a Clinician and What Does He Do?" Speech to Johns Hopkins medical students, reprinted in *The New England Journal of Medicine* 283, (1970).

[2] Cheshire Calhoun, "The Virtue of Civility," *Philosophy & Public Affairs* 29, no. 3 (2000).

[3] Judith Martin, *Miss Manners Rescues Civilization* (New York: Crown Publishing, 1996).

[4] Ibid.

[5] Ibid.

Chapter Three

1. Sarah Buss, "Appearing Respectful: The Moral Significance of Manners," *Ethics* 109, no. 4 (1999), 795-826.
2. Matthew Wynia, Stephen Latham, Audiey Kao, Jessica Berg, Linda Emanuel, "Medical Professionalism in Society," *New England Journal of Medicine* 341 (1999).
3. Sarah Buss, "Appearing Respectful," *Ethics* (1999).
4. Ibid.
5. Philip Tumulty, "The Art of Healing," *Johns Hopkins Medical Journal* 143 (1978).
6. George Beller, "President's Page: Patient Satisfaction: A personal perspective," *Journal of American College Cardiology* 37 (2001).
7. David Pendleton, Theo Schofield, Peter Tate, and Peter Havelock, *The New Consultation: Developing Doctor-Patient Communication* (Oxford: Oxford University Press, 2003).
8. Howard Beckman and Richard Frankel, "The Effect of Physician Behavior on the Collection of Data," *Annals of Internal Medicine* 101 (1984).
9. Jerome Groopman, *How Doctors Think* (Boston: Houghton Mifflin Company, 2007).
10. Lewis Thomas, *The Youngest Science—Notes of a Medicine Watcher* (New York: The Viking Press, 1983).

[11] Bernard Lown, *The Lost Art of Healing* (Boston: Houghton Mifflin Company, 1996).
[12] Calhoun, Cheshire, "Expecting Common Decency." *Philosophy of Education* (2002), 28–35, http://ojs.ed.uiuc.edu/index.php/pes/article/viewFile/1789/499. Accessed Mar 30, 2011.
[13] W. T. Branch Jr., R. Frankel, C. F. Gracey, et al. "A good Clinician and a caring person: Longitudinal Faculty Development and the Enhancement of the Human Dimension of Care." *Academic Medicine* 84, no. 1 (2009), 117–25.
[14] Michael Kahn, "Etiquette-Based Medicine," *New England Journal of Medicine* 358 (2008).

Chapter Four

[1] Jerome Groopman, *How Doctors Think* (Chicago: Mariner Books, 2007).
[2] Francis Peabody, *Doctor and Patient: Papers on the Relationship of the Physician to Men and Institutions* (New York: Macmillan Company, 1930).
[3] Judith Martin, *Miss Manners' Guide to Excruciatingly Correct Behavior* (New York: W. W. Norton and Company, 2005).
[4] Sharon Schwarze, "Being On Time for Appointments," *Journal of Clinical Ethics* 3, no. 140 (1992).

⁵ Barbara Korsch, "What do Patients and Parents Want to Know? What do They Need to Know?" *Pediatrics* 74 (1984).
⁶ Glen Elwyn, A. Edwards, P. Kinnersley, "Shared Decision Making in Primary Care: the Neglected Second Half of the Consultation," *British Journal of General Practice* 49 (1999), 477–82.
⁷ Ibid.

Chapter Five

¹ Sentinel Event Alert, "Behaviors that undermine a culture of safety," The Joint Commission, Issue 40 (2008), http://www.jointcommission.org/assets/1/18/SEA_40.PDF. Accessed June 9, 2011.
² Ibid.

Chapter Six

¹ American Academy of Pediatrics, "Your Child's Health Record" (2009), https://www.nfaap.org/netforum/eweb/DynamicPage.aspx?webcode=aapbks_productdetail&key=9e3548a6-ed9e-40ca-9857-799d81e3b5f7#.
² CDC Vaccines and Immunizations, "Polio Disease: Questions and Answers," http://www.cdc.gov/vaccines/vpd-vac/polio/dis-faqs.htm. Accessed October 27, 2011.

About the Authors

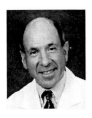
Barry Silverman, MD is a fellow in the American College of Physicians, a fellow in the American College of Cardiology, a member of the American Osler Society, Clinical Assistant Professor of Medicine at Emory University Medical School, and the editor of *Atlanta Medicine*.

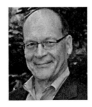
Saul Adler, MD is a fellow of the American Academy of Pediatrics. He is an assistant editor for *Narrative*, the digital literary magazine.